## Acclaim for *It Starts with the Egg*

"Rebecca Fett's stellar constellation of perspective, experience, knowledge, and scientific background may well revolutionize our current global conversation, understanding and practices related to fertility...It is hard to overestimate the impact that this book may have on the lives of many."

DR. CLAUDIA WELCH, AUTHOR OF *BALANCE YOUR HORMONES, BALANCE YOUR LIFE*.

"With detailed, up to date research Rebecca Fett provides a clear, cool-headed guide to both the science that determines IVF success, and the practical changes that patients can make to drastically increase their chances of IVF success."

—DR. LINDSAY WU, LABORATORY FOR AGEING RESEARCH, UNIVERSITY OF NEW SOUTH WALES MEDICAL CENTER, AUSTRALIA.

"This is a very useful resource: well-researched, accessibly written and with easy to follow take-home messages and action plans. I would recommend this to any woman who is trying to conceive."

—DR. CLAIRE DEAKIN, UNIVERSITY COLLEGE LONDON, INSTITUTE OF CHILD HEALTH.

"A thoroughly-researched and eye-opening account of how small, simple lifestyle changes can have powerful, positive effects on your health and fertility. A must-read for women wanting the best chance of conceiving a healthy baby."

—BETH GREER, BESTSELLING AUTHOR OF *SUPER NATURAL HOME*.

"It Starts with the Egg presents a reasoned and balanced review of the latest science linking environmental chemicals to reduced fertility and other health problems. Readers will find sound advice for how to avoid chemicals of concern, providing a useful guide for couples that want to improve their chances of a healthy pregnancy."

—DR. LAURA VANDENBERG, UNIVERSITY OF MASSACHUSETTS, AMHERST, SCHOOL OF PUBLIC HEALTH.

"This timely synthesis of scientific literature is essential reading for both women and men wanting practical, evidence-based recommendations to enhance their fertility."

—DR. LORETTA MCKINNON, EPIDEMIOLOGIST, PRINCESS ALEXANDRA HOSPITAL.

"With 'It Starts with the Egg,' Rebecca Fett delivers a much needed overview on the available scientific evidence regarding the influence of nutrition on fertility and fertility treatment, providing a valuable resource for couples trying to conceive."

—DR. JOHN TWIGT, DEPARTMENT OF OBSTETRICS AND GYNECOLOGY, ERASMUS MEDICAL CENTER, NETHERLANDS.

"Rebecca has done a great service for all women, children, and future generations by starting at the beginning of a human life and examining which toxic chemicals cause harm to the egg...This book is a wonderful addition to the growing library of information on toxic exposures."

—DEBRA LYNN DADD, AUTHOR OF TOXIC FREE: HOW TO PROTECT YOUR HEALTH AND HOME FROM THE CHEMICALS THAT ARE MAKING YOU SICK

"Rebecca Fett did a stellar job of researching and summarizing the current understanding of the impact of egg quality on IVF pregnancy chances. "

—DR. NORBERT GLEICHER, REPRODUCTIVE ENDOCRINOLOGIST, THE CENTER FOR HUMAN REPRODUCTION, NEW YORK.

"Rebecca Fett's 'It Starts with the Egg' is a complete guide to everything a woman can do to improve her egg quality before trying to conceive..."It Starts with the Egg" also breaks information down in easy-to-digest bullet points that show exactly what to do to get to where you want to be: the parent of a happy, healthy, gorgeous baby."

—CHERYL ALKON, AUTHOR OF BALANCING PREGNANCY WITH PRE-EXISTING DIABETES: HEALTHY MOM, HEALTHY BABY.

How the **Science of Egg Quality** Can Help You
**Get Pregnant Naturally, Prevent Miscarriage,**
and **Improve Your Odds in IVF**

Second Edition

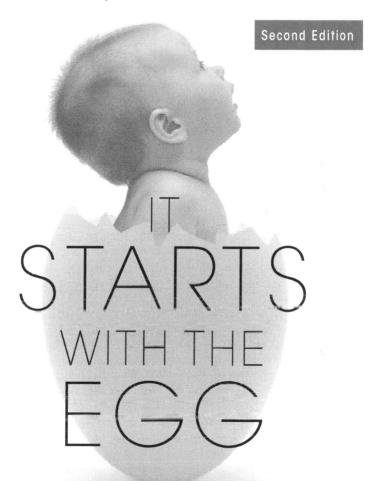

IT
STARTS
WITH THE
EGG

REBECCA FETT

Franklin Fox Publishing
New York

FRANKLIN FOX PUBLISHING

First edition: © 2014 by Rebecca Fett
Second edition: © 2019 by Rebecca Fett

Published in the United States by Franklin Fox Publishing LLC, New
York.
Interior/cover design: Steven Plummer/ SPDesign
Front Cover Photo: Tsekhmister
Back Cover Photo: Tessa Falk

This book is intended to provide helpful and informative material. It is
not intended to provide medical advice and cannot replace the advice
of a medical professional. The reader should consult his or her doctor
before adopting any of the suggestions in this book. The author and
publisher specifically disclaim all responsibility for any liability, loss,
or risk, personal or otherwise, which is incurred as a consequence of
the use and application of any of the contents of this book.

ISBN-13: 9780999676189
ISBN-10: 0999676180

www.itstartswiththeegg.com

# Table of Contents

In a broader sense, *It Starts with the Egg* has had a greater impact than I ever could have imagined. Each year, more than 30,000 women are reading the book and putting the advice into action. Many of the supplements described, such as Coenzyme Q10 and DHEA, are now widely recommended by top IVF clinics. At the same time, the tendency for women to take a variety of unproven and potentially harmful herbal supplements is falling out of favor. It is now also becoming standard practice for women preparing for IVF to take steps to reduce exposure to hormone-disrupting toxins such as BPA and phthalates, a topic that was previously neglected in standard fertility advice.

Yet I have to admit that the book has also caused some women to become overly stressed by trying to avoid every possible source of hormone-disrupting toxins. The original impetus for this second edition was my hope to address this problem by clarifying what to focus on and re-emphasizing that complete avoidance is not the goal. Instead, the aim is to make a few simple changes to avoid the worst offenders, in order to ensure that you do not have an unusually high level of exposure to the particular toxins that have the most impact on fertility.

The latest research on BPA and phthalates, discussed in this new edition, lends further support to the notion that it is only higher than average levels that we need to be concerned about. This new research also provides greater guidance on where to focus our efforts, so we can be less worried about potential toxin sources that make very little difference.

New studies also further illuminate the supplement and

dietary advice in the chapters that follow. For example, studies have confirmed that the approach of emphasizing blood sugar control and adopting a Mediterranean-style diet truly can improve IVF success rates. Additional studies published since the first edition also provide much stronger evidence for many of the supplements discussed, such as DHEA.

With the benefit of several randomized clinical studies, it is now beyond controversy that DHEA can improve the number and quality of eggs in women with diminished ovarian reserve.

Likewise, there is now more science than ever before on how to improve sperm quality, and just how important this is. Recent studies have confirmed that sperm quality is likely a key contributor to the risk of pregnancy loss. Yet the research has also brought good news on this front, with randomized controlled studies demonstrating that supplements such as omega-3 fish oil can help correct the specific aspects of sperm quality that contribute to pregnancy loss. This new edition explains all of this latest science and more, to give you the best possible chance of conceiving and having a healthy pregnancy.

complex system in which chromosomes in an egg are recombined and then mechanically separated before and after fertilization. As I delved deeper into the scientific papers addressing egg quality, all the pieces that I had learned about years earlier started to fit together with groundbreaking recent studies to form a picture of the various causes of chromosomal abnormalities in eggs and the influence of external factors. In short, the research revealed a quiet revolution in the way we think about egg quality.

I started putting into practice everything I had learned. I improved my diet by cutting out refined carbohydrates (to lower insulin, which is shown to impact egg quality), started taking a small handful of daily supplements, and took extra steps to limit my exposure to household toxins, such as replacing plastic with glass and buying fragrance-free cleaning products.

I also decided to take the hormone DHEA, which, as I will explain later in this book, has now been shown in numerous clinical trials to improve the chance of success for those with diminished ovarian reserve.

During those months, I started thinking of myself as "prepregnant" and protected my eggs the way I would protect a growing baby if I were pregnant. I found it reassuring that even if this particular IVF cycle failed, I could at least take comfort in the knowledge that I had done absolutely everything I could to make healthy embryos.

That said, I was not expecting any miracles. I still suspected that with a diminished reserve of eggs, I had an uphill battle. I had seen the statistics showing IVF success rates in relation to ovarian reserve, and they were not grounds for optimism.

A couple of months after beginning my quest for egg quality, my husband and I went back to the fertility clinic for a routine check of my ovaries before starting the IVF stimulation medication. We were shocked to witness how much had changed. Instead of a couple of follicles (the small structures in which a single egg matures) in each ovary, the ultrasound showed that I probably had about 20 eggs maturing. This number was perfectly normal, and I felt the weight of the words "diminished ovarian reserve" lifting from my shoulders. Our odds had suddenly become a lot better.

Nevertheless, I remained nervous. The weeks passed, and each day became a routine of injections, pills, ultrasounds, and blood tests. The tests gave us every reason to expect a good outcome, but as our doctor explained, there are never any guarantees in an IVF cycle because so much can go wrong. Every morning and evening when I took out my boxes of syringes, needles, and vials of expensive fertility drugs, preparing to give myself several injections, I felt a twinge of anxiety, knowing this could all be for nothing.

On the day of the egg retrieval, I woke up after the procedure to discover that they had retrieved 22 eggs, and all were mature. Even through the haze of the anesthetic, this news brought huge relief. I tried not to get too excited, knowing there were still quite a few hurdles to go, but suddenly we were faced with the very real prospect that this cycle could actually work.

At this point, I knew it was a numbers game. In a typical IVF cycle where 20 eggs are retrieved, approximately 15 will fertilize. Of those embryos, only a third are likely to make it to five-day-old embryos ready to be transferred into the uterus.

We planned to do a single embryo transfer, so we needed just one good-quality embryo that made it to this critical five-day-old "blastocyst" stage. But knowing that a huge proportion of embryo transfers fail and that we might need to do a second or third round of embryo transfer to become pregnant, the more embryos we could get, the better.

Later that day, after we waited to find out how many eggs had fertilized, the clinic called. Out of 22 eggs, 19 had fertilized. There was now a very good chance that a few embryos would make it to the blastocyst stage, although many couples in the same position are not so lucky. Five days later, we were in for another surprise. Every single one of our embryos had survived to become a good-quality blastocyst. This result was simply unheard of. In fact, even though our clinic had treated thousands of patients and had one of the highest success rates in the United States, we had easily set a new clinic record for the number of good-quality blastocysts from a single cycle.

On the sixth day after the egg retrieval, we transferred one perfect-looking embryo and began the notoriously difficult two-week wait to find out if our surrogate was pregnant. What happened next was what we all wish for: a positive pregnancy test. It is impossible to know if the same result would have happened without my mission to improve my egg quality, but the scientific research shows that egg quality is the single most important factor in determining whether an egg will fertilize and survive to the blastocyst stage. It also determines whether an embryo is capable of implanting and leading to a viable pregnancy.

As I told this story to my female friends, the reaction was the same, regardless of the life stage they were in. Everyone wanted to know what they could do to improve their own chances. I found myself wanting to delve into the scientific research again. It is one thing to make a determination for myself on whether the research shows that a particular supplement is safe and worthwhile, but if I was going to share my knowledge with other women who were trying to get pregnant or who had suffered multiple miscarriages, I had a much greater responsibility to get it right. And so I began an even more exhaustive search and analysis of the latest research relating to egg quality.

I carefully analyzed hundreds of scientific papers investigating specific effects of toxins and nutrients on biological processes, identifying influences on fertility and miscarriage rates in large, population-based studies, and uncovering the factors that influence success rates in IVF. (You can find these scientific papers listed in the references section, along with information on how to access them online.) This comprehensive research was an undertaking most fertility specialists are simply too busy to do, and, unsurprisingly, many doctors are not up to date on recent findings.

I quickly learned that the standard advice of IVF clinics and fertility books was not keeping pace with research. At that time, in 2013, no one was talking about the new research showing that BPA has a significant negative effect on fertility and IVF success rates. DHEA was considered highly controversial, and clinics were simply not telling their patients about it.

Even now, these and other issues are often overlooked, and many doctors just do not have the time to keep up with every relevant area of research. As one example, there were several studies published in 2017 and 2018 finding that for the purpose of preventing miscarriage, the optimal vitamin D level is much higher than previously thought. Yet many doctors still follow old guidelines for vitamin D levels that are based on preserving bone health.

This is not to suggest that all IVF clinics are behind the times when it comes to research on supplements and egg quality. Some do stay abreast of the research and recommend a cocktail of supplements that closely aligns with the advice in this book. But these clinics generally do not explain the fascinating story of how each supplement is thought to work and cannot reach patients outside the IVF context. They also fail to mention all the important measures you can take other than supplements.

Many women preparing for IVF are aware that they may not be getting the most up-to-date advice about what supplements can improve their chances, and so turn to the internet for information. This path often leads to supplements that are not supported by any scientific research or that may actually be harmful for egg quality, such as royal jelly and L-arginine. This book not only discusses the measures that may help but also debunks myths about some supplements that may do more harm than good.

For women trying to conceive naturally instead of through IVF, relying on internet research to figure out which supplements to take can be particularly problematic because egg quality is not the only issue to consider.

As just one example, research has clearly demonstrated that melatonin supplements improve egg quality and are thus often recommended for women undergoing IVF. But the problem is that taking melatonin supplements long term could potentially disrupt ovulation. This means that melatonin is only helpful in the IVF context, where natural regulation of ovulation is less important. If you are trying to conceive naturally, disrupted ovulation is a significant problem, and taking melatonin could actually make it more difficult to get pregnant. Trawling the internet for ideas on what to take for fertility is likely to miss these nuances and cause trouble for many women.

The supplement DHEA provides another example of some of the problems with the standard advice of many IVF clinics. If you have been diagnosed with diminished ovarian reserve and are preparing for IVF, whether or not you will be advised to take DHEA depends more on which IVF clinic you happen to be attending rather than any logical basis. Many clinics also leave the decision of whether to take DHEA up to the individual patient, without performing any testing or providing any detailed information about the strength of the clinical evidence. We deserve better and have a right to make truly informed decisions.

Seeing the immense gap between the research and conventional fertility advice, I felt compelled to help by distilling the clinical research into concrete, comprehensible information. As I became more convinced of the impact of external factors on egg quality and how important egg quality is to the chance of conceiving, whether naturally or through IVF, I felt an urgent need to help educate other women struggling with infertility. And so this book was born.

Seeing our growing baby on the 12-week ultrasound and hearing the heartbeat were moments of such pure joy that I wanted the same for everyone else going through the process of fertility treatment or planning to have a baby. Of course, in the world of infertility there are never any promises. No one can offer a guaranteed way to get pregnant because there are so many variables and unique challenges, particularly if you are trying to conceive after the age of 35. But this book offers a plan to improve your odds and in doing so, improve your overall health and prepare your body for a healthy pregnancy.

## How to Use this Book

### If you are just starting out

If you have just begun trying to get pregnant and have no reason to expect fertility challenges, you will likely not need to adopt every suggestion in this book. By following the supplement recommendations in the *basic plan* (summarized in chapter 12), starting to reduce some of the worst offenders when it comes to hormone-disrupting toxins, and shifting your diet slightly along the lines discussed in chapter 13, you may be able to get pregnant faster and reduce the risk of miscarriage.

Improving egg quality is helpful even without any specific fertility concern because even young, healthy women have a significant proportion of abnormal eggs. If the eggs you happen to ovulate for a few months in a row are affected, this will increase the time it takes you to conceive and put you at risk of losing a pregnancy. Many of the recommendations in this book are also beneficial for your overall health and the health of your future baby.

## If you are having difficulty conceiving

If you have been trying to conceive for some time but have not yet moved on to fertility treatments such as IVF, you can follow the supplement advice in the *intermediate plan*. This plan adds a small number of additional supplements to support egg quality, with an emphasis on antioxidants. (See chapters 6 and 7 for a detailed explanation and chapter 12 for a summary of the supplement recommendations.)

The intermediate plan will be slightly modified for those with polycystic ovary syndrome (PCOS), to incorporate supplements that have been specifically found to improve fertility in that context.

## If you are trying to conceive through IVF or IUI

If you have been battling infertility for a substantial length of time and are trying to conceive with assisted reproduction techniques such as IVF, you have the most to gain from a comprehensive approach to improving egg quality. This includes strategies to minimize toxin exposure, dietary changes, and the supplements included in the *advanced plan*. These supplements are intended to help those with age-related infertility, endometriosis, diminished ovarian reserve, or the catch-all diagnosis of unexplained infertility. The precise supplements that are most helpful for each situation are discussed in chapters 6 through 11, with chapter 12 providing an example of an overall supplement plan.

As the next chapter explains, poor egg quality is often the culprit in women with unexplained infertility. The rapid decline in fertility that begins in the mid-30s is also largely a product of declining egg quality, and this often becomes a limiting factor to becoming pregnant, even with the assistance of IVF. The success rates in IVF cycles are very much dependent on age.[1] Unless donor eggs are used, IVF can only do so much.

Whether your infertility is unexplained or has been put down to age, endometriosis, or diminished ovarian reserve, improving your egg quality should be your primary focus in trying to conceive. Research shows that only good-quality eggs are likely to become good-quality embryos that can survive the critical first week and successfully implant to result in a pregnancy. It is therefore critical that you maximize the number of good-quality eggs that have the potential to become a healthy baby.

## Recurrent miscarriage

Improving egg and sperm quality could also play an important role in preventing miscarriages. In some cases, recurrent miscarriage is caused by clotting or immune factors. Another common cause is an underactive thyroid gland.[2] By finding out if you have one of these medical causes of miscarriage, which explain about a quarter of miscarriages, you may be able to reduce the chance of it happening again.

For example, in women who have antibodies attacking their thyroid (known as Hashimoto's thyroiditis), treatment with an added thyroid hormone called levothyroxine reduces the miscarriage rate by more than 50 percent.[3] (For more information on testing and treatment for the various medical causes of miscarriage, I recommend reading *Not Broken* by Dr. Lora Shahine, a reproductive endocrinologist who specializes in recurrent miscarriage.)

If testing rules out clotting, immune, or thyroid problems

as the cause of your pregnancy losses, the most likely culprit is egg quality. This is because a poor-quality egg with chromosomal abnormalities will develop into an embryo and then fetus with chromosomal abnormalities and very little chance of surviving. Chromosomal abnormalities are in fact the most common cause of early miscarriage, accounting for 40–50 percent of miscarriages.[4]

As the next chapter explains, these chromosomal abnormalities often originate in the egg and become even more frequent with age.[5] In this book, you will learn how chromosomal abnormalities often occur during the last phase of egg maturation before ovulation and what you can do to reduce the chance of your next pregnancy being affected. New research is also showing that sperm quality can be a major contributor to miscarriage, likely by raising the risk of chromosomal abnormalities.

If you have had two or more miscarriages and your doctor cannot find a medical cause, or you know that chromosomal abnormalities affected your previous pregnancies (such as Down syndrome or another "trisomy"), consider following the *advanced plan* for at least three months before trying to conceive again. See chapter 12 for a summary of the supplement recommendations for this plan.

This updated edition also provides additional information on specific supplements and dietary strategies that may be most helpful for those with a history of miscarriage driven by immune factors or inflammation. (See, for example, chapters 6 and 7, and the specific dietary recommendations toward the end of chapter 13.)

## What About the Sperm?

While the focus of this book is egg quality, many of the same external factors impact sperm in a similar way, as discussed in chapter 14. Although often overlooked, sperm quality can in some cases have a significant effect on your likelihood of conceiving and carrying to term. It is time to rethink the assumption that the father's age and lifestyle factors are irrelevant. If you know or suspect that male factor infertility is part of your challenge in conceiving, or you have a history of recurrent pregnancy loss, it will be particularly valuable to apply the recommendations in chapter 14, which explains the specific nutrients that affect sperm quality. Even if you have no cause for concern about sperm quality, you will learn why it is important for all men trying to conceive to take certain supplements to increase the chance of success.

## Conclusion

Whether you are trying to conceive naturally, pursuing IVF, or trying again after a pregnancy loss, it is imperative that you do what you can to improve your egg quality. It takes approximately three months for an immature egg to develop into a mature egg ready for ovulation, and this is the crucial window of time. In subsequent chapters, you will learn the most important things you can do, but to understand how these lifestyle factors can improve egg quality, it is necessary to first understand what egg quality means and how chromosomal abnormalities occur. That is the subject of chapter 1.

# Part 1

# THE SCIENCE OF
# EGG QUALITY

# CHAPTER 1

# Understanding Egg Quality

*"When you know better you do better."*
—MAYA ANGELOU

THE DECLINE IN fertility as we age is almost entirely a result of the decline in egg quantity and quality. We know this because older women who use donor eggs have pregnancy rates similar to younger women. But what does egg quality mean? Broadly, it describes the potential of an egg to become a viable pregnancy after fertilization. And this is no trivial matter—the vast majority of fertilized eggs simply do not have what it takes.

## Egg Quality Is Everything

For any embryo, the first few weeks after fertilization represent a major hurdle, and many embryos stop developing at some point during this time. In fact, most naturally conceived

studies were investigating miscarriages from recognized pregnancies only, and the rate of chromosomal abnormalities is likely to be much higher for losses that occur in the short time after fertilization.[9]

A common reaction to this information is that chromosomal errors in eggs are beyond our control, but recent scientific research is showing that is not true. The proportion of eggs with chromosomal abnormalities can be influenced by nutrients and lifestyle factors you can control. As will be discussed later in this chapter, research suggests that one way external factors can influence egg quality is by boosting or compromising the egg's potential to produce energy at critical times—energy that provides the fuel for proper chromosome processing.

The best-known example of a chromosomal abnormality originating in the egg is Down syndrome, which becomes much more common as women age and egg quality declines. In 95 percent of cases, Down syndrome is caused by the egg providing an extra copy of chromosome 21, which results in the fetus having three copies instead of the usual two.[10] For this reason, Down syndrome is also called trisomy 21.

Down syndrome is just one example of a chromosomal abnormality, but it is perhaps the best known because it is one of the few in which the affected fetus can survive to term. Some babies with trisomy 13 or trisomy 18 (an extra copy of chromosome 13 or 18) can also survive to term, but with life-threatening medical problems. An extra copy of other chromosomes will prevent the embryo from developing past the first few days or weeks, or will cause an early miscarriage.[11] This is why we rarely hear about chromosomal errors involving extra copies of these other chromosomes, even though they are very common.

While having an extra copy of a chromosome is the most common type of chromosomal abnormality, occasionally a missing chromosome or more complex errors can also occur.

An egg with the incorrect number of chromosomes is called "aneuploid." An embryo created from an aneuploid egg will also be aneuploid and will have very little potential to successfully implant in the uterus. Even when aneuploid embryos are able to progress to a pregnancy, the vast majority of such pregnancies end in an early miscarriage.[12]

In women over 40, more than half of their eggs may be chromosomally abnormal.[13] In fact, by some measures, the rate of abnormalities in women over 40 is as high as 70–80 percent.[14] Studying chromosomal abnormalities in eggs, we see an exponential increase in the fertility challenge faced with age, starting in the mid- to late thirties. But egg quality has an impact in all age groups, and chromosomal errors in younger women are much more common than you might expect.

Even in women under 35, up to a quarter of eggs are aneuploid, on average.[15] This means that if you are a young, healthy woman without any fertility issues, there will still be many ovulation cycles in which you have little potential to conceive. If the egg that you ovulate in a given month is chromosomally abnormal and unable to support a pregnancy, using ovulation prediction kits and charts to achieve fertilization with perfect timing will not make any difference; you will probably not be able to conceive until the next cycle in which you ovulate a good egg.

The dramatic impact of chromosomal abnormalities on the chance of conceiving and carrying to term is particularly apparent in the IVF context. If this factor is taken out of the equation, the pregnancy rates skyrocket. We know this from a process called Preimplantation Genetic Screening (or PGS), in which embryos are first screened for abnormalities in every chromosome and only the normal embryos are transferred.

This is very different from the traditional measure of "embryo quality" in the IVF context, which is based on the growth rate and overall appearance of the embryo. A slow-growing embryo with irregular-looking cells is less likely to lead to a pregnancy, but it has become clear in recent years that assessment of embryo quality based on appearance or "morphology" is no guarantee. What matters much more is screening for embryos that have normal chromosomes.

When comprehensive chromosome screening was introduced for poor-prognosis patients at a leading IVF clinic in 2010, the difference was dramatic. Instead of the usual 13 percent of transferred embryos successfully implanting for patients 41–42 years old, selecting only chromosomally normal embryos boosted the implantation rate to 38 percent. As a result, the proportion of women in this age group completing an IVF cycle who actually took home a baby *doubled*.[16]

The technique of comprehensive chromosome screening to identify the best embryos was pioneered at the Colorado Center for Reproductive Medicine (CCRM) by Dr. William Schoolcraft, a highly regarded fertility specialist and the author of several studies showing the success of this approach.

Dr. Schoolcraft's studies include many examples of individual patients who were able to conceive only after chromosomally normal embryos were chosen for transfer.[17] One patient mentioned in Dr. Schoolcraft's 2009 study was a 37-year-old who had gone through six previous IVF cycles in which the transferred embryos did not implant. She then began yet another IVF cycle, this time with chromosomal screening on 10 of her embryos. Out of those 10 embryos, seven were found to be chromosomally abnormal. If screening had not been done and embryos had been chosen for transfer by appearance alone, there would have been a high probability of transferring chromosomally abnormal embryos. Those embryos would most likely have failed to implant or led to a miscarriage. Instead of taking that chance, her doctors transferred the three chromosomally normal embryos, and she became pregnant with twins.

Another patient in Dr. Schoolcraft's study was a 33-year-old woman who had suffered six miscarriages. In her next IVF cycle, chromosomal screening revealed that out of 11 embryos, eight had chromosomal errors. Without screening, there was a good chance that one of the eight abnormal embryos would have been transferred, likely resulting in no pregnancy or a seventh miscarriage. Instead, her doctors were able to select two chromosomally normal embryos, and she gave birth to twins.

Sometimes chromosomal screening reveals just how heavily the odds can be stacked against a successful pregnancy. This is apparent in Dr. Schoolcraft's example of a 41-year-old woman who was able to conceive after chromosomal screening identified the single embryo out of eight that was chromosomally normal and had the potential for a normal, healthy pregnancy.

While chromosomal screening represents a very significant

advance, it is not a cure-all. One of the main problems is that screening may show that none of the embryos created in an IVF cycle are chromosomally normal. As a result, there will be no good embryo available to transfer. This happened to about a third of patients in one study,[18] demonstrating that egg quality will still remain a limiting factor to becoming pregnant, even with preimplantation screening.

Yet chromosomal screening does hold great promise and shows the dramatic impact of egg and embryo quality on pregnancy rates. Interestingly, this impact is not limited to "poor-prognosis patients." A group in Japan set out to determine how much they could improve pregnancy rates in IVF cycles by choosing to transfer only chromosomally normal embryos, but this time they were looking at women under 35 with a good prognosis and no previous miscarriages.[19] In the control group, in which embryos were chosen by appearance alone, 41 percent of patients became pregnant per IVF cycle and carried to at least 20 weeks. In the group in which embryos were chosen by chromosomal screening, the pregnancy rate jumped to 69 percent. The miscarriage rates were also very different: 9 percent in the control group and just 2.6 percent in the screened group.

The lesson we can take away from the positive results of chromosomal screening is that having a chromosomally normal embryo has a huge impact on the chance of a successful pregnancy, no matter how you are trying to conceive. Even if trying to conceive naturally, your chance of becoming pregnant and carrying to term is very much determined by your egg quality. Luckily, egg quality is not entirely predetermined by your age or fixed in time. It can change.

There is, in fact, an enormous variation in chromosomal abnormality rates between different women of the same age.[20] One 35-year-old may ovulate very few chromosomally normal eggs over a given time frame, while another woman's eggs may all be normal at the same age. This was shown in a study of IVF patients in Germany and Italy in which the percentage of chromosomally normal eggs ranged greatly between different women of the same age. The number of normal eggs also varied widely over time for each woman, which was seen as a significant difference in the proportion of normal eggs between two consecutive IVF cycles. The researchers described the variation over time and between different women as random and unpredictable, but only because they did not connect their research to the many other studies showing specific influences on the rates of chromosomal abnormalities. The fascinating research discussed in the remainder of this book establishes that this variability is not purely random; on the contrary, a wide range of external factors impact egg quality.

Countless clinical studies have shown that avoiding certain toxins and adding specific supplements can increase the percentage of eggs that can develop into a good-quality embryo, increase the percentage of embryos that implant in the uterus, and reduce the risk of early-pregnancy loss. There is strong scientific evidence that some of these improvements are due to a reduction in the proportion of eggs with chromosomal abnormalities, confirming the fact that egg quality is something we have the power to change.

## How Do Eggs Become
## "Chromosomally Abnormal"?

The process of egg production is very long and error-prone. The development of each egg begins before a woman is even born, in the newly forming ovaries during the first trimester of pregnancy. A girl is born with all the eggs she will ever have, and each egg exists in a state of suspended animation until a few months before ovulation.

Approximately four months before ovulation, a small pool of immature eggs begin to grow, and while most will die off naturally, one lead egg is selected from the pool to finish maturing.[21] The fully grown egg completes ovulation by bursting from its follicle and traveling down the fallopian tube, ready to be fertilized.

During the decades-long interval between early egg development and ovulation, eggs have many opportunities to accumulate damage as a part of normal aging. The traditional belief is that by the time a woman is 40, her eggs have already accumulated chromosomal abnormalities, and nothing can be done to change that. But that is not scientifically correct, because most chromosomal errors actually occur shortly before ovulation, in later stages of a process called "meiosis."

An egg ends up with the incorrect number of chromosomes when meiosis goes awry. Meiosis involves carefully aligning chromosome copies along the middle of the egg, then pulling one set to each end of the egg with a network of microscopic tubules. One set of chromosomes is then pushed out of the egg in what is called a "polar body." A developing egg actually does this twice—it starts out with four copies of each chromosome and, if the process goes correctly, ends up with just one copy of each chromosome.

If this process fails at any stage, the end result is an extra or missing copy of a chromosome. Although the first round of meiosis begins before a girl is born, most of the chromosomal processing activity happens in the months immediately before an egg is ovulated.

The critical point to note—and a point that many fertility doctors are not aware of—is that most of the chromosomal abnormalities in eggs do not accumulate gradually over 30 or 40 years as an egg ages, but instead happen in the couple of months before an egg is ovulated. In other words, aging does not directly cause chromosomal abnormalities; rather, it creates conditions that predispose eggs to mature incorrectly shortly before ovulation.[22]

This means that by changing those conditions before ovulation, you can increase the odds of an egg maturing with the correct number of chromosomes. In short, you may be able to influence the quality of eggs that you ovulate a couple of months from now because chromosomal errors in those eggs have probably not occurred yet.

This leads us to the fundamental issue: How can an egg be predisposed to mature with an incorrect number of chromosomes, and what can you do about it? Every chapter in this book addresses different aspects of that question, but a common theme is the egg's energy supply.

## Energy Production in the Egg

It takes an enormous amount of energy for the egg to process chromosomes correctly and do all the other work necessary to mature properly. It turns out that the energy-producing structures inside eggs change significantly with age and in response to nutrients and other external factors.[23] These structures, called "mitochondria," are found in nearly every cell in the body. They act as miniature power plants to transform various fuel sources into energy that the cell can use, in the form of ATP.

ATP is quite literally the energy of life. It moves muscles, makes enzymes work, and powers nerve impulses. Just about every other biological process depends on it. And it is the primary form of energy used by eggs. A growing egg needs a lot of ATP and has a lot of mitochondria. In fact, each egg has more than fifteen thousand mitochondria—over ten times more than any other cell in the body.[24] The follicle cells surrounding the egg also contain many mitochondria and supply the egg with additional ATP.[25] But these mitochondria must be in good condition to make enough energy.

Over time, and in response to oxidative stress (explained in chapter 6), mitochondria become damaged and less able to produce energy.[26] Without sufficient energy, egg and embryo development may go awry or stop altogether.[27] As explained by Dr. Robert Casper, a leading fertility specialist in Toronto, "the ageing female reproductive system is like a forgotten flashlight on the top shelf of a closet. When you stumble across it a few years later and try to switch it on, it won't work, not because there's anything wrong with the flashlight but because the batteries inside it have died."[28]

A growing body of evidence suggests that the ability of an egg to produce energy when needed is critically important to being able to mature with the correct number of chromosomes.

It is also vital to an embryo's potential to survive the first week and successfully implant.

Poorly functioning mitochondria may be one of the most important reasons some women's eggs are more likely to end up with chromosomal abnormalities or otherwise lack the potential to become a viable embryo. What you can do to help "recharge" your mitochondria and thereby boost your eggs' energy supply is the subject of several chapters later in this book, but first we turn to another contributor to chromosomal errors in developing eggs—the toxin BPA.

# CHAPTER 2

# How BPA Impacts Fertility

*"The most exciting phrase to hear in science, the one that heralds new discoveries, is not 'Eureka!' (I found it!) but 'That's funny...'"*

— ISAAC ASIMOV

I F YOU WANT the best possible chance of becoming pregnant and delivering a healthy baby, one of the first steps you should take is to reduce your exposure to specific toxins that can harm fertility. This subject has long been neglected in traditional fertility books and in doctors' offices, but it is incredibly important to learn about if you are trying to conceive.

One toxin that has been proven to compromise egg quality and fertility is BPA, which stands for bisphenol A. This chemical is still commonly used in everything from plastic food containers to paper receipts, despite years of public attention about its potential health dangers.

This chapter will arm you with the resources you need to minimize your exposure to BPA—illustrating how small, simple changes can have powerful positive effects on your health and fertility.

## Where We Are

When *It Starts with the Egg* was first published in 2014, the concept of minimizing BPA exposure in order to safeguard egg quality was relatively new. The first edition of this book therefore focused on persuading people to adopt this radical new mindset, with the unfortunate consequence that many readers became overly stressed about avoiding every possible source of BPA.

Now the need to minimize BPA is no longer controversial and most women preparing for IVF generally accept that it is best to replace their reusable plastic water bottle and food containers with glass or stainless steel. It is now time to focus on the most important message: that our goal is to reduce our exposure, not to avoid BPA completely. As this chapter explains, the most recent studies indicate that the real concern with BPA arises when women have above-average levels. The good news is that you can easily reduce your exposure once you know how. But first, a brief overview of how we got here and the current state of the evidence.

## How It All Began

The story of BPA and fertility begins with a chance discovery so unexpected that researchers spent years verifying their results before going public. Dr. Patricia Hunt and her research

group at Case Western Reserve University were using laboratory mice to study egg development and saw something very
unusual in August 1998: a dramatic increase in the number of
chromosomally abnormal eggs. In mice, typically only 1–2 percent of eggs are unable to properly align the chromosomes in
the middle of the egg. However, in Dr. Hunt's laboratory, this
specific problem suddenly spiked and affected 40 percent of the
eggs, along with other severe chromosomal aberrations. When
the eggs matured, they were much more likely to have an incorrect number of chromosomes. As Dr. Hunt observed, "I was
really horrified because we saw this night and day change."[1]

The researchers began a thorough investigation and eventually found the culprit. BPA had started leaching out of the
mice's plastic cages and water bottles after they were washed
with detergent. When all of these damaged plastic cages and
bottles were replaced, the rate of eggs with chromosomal
errors began to return to normal. Dr. Hunt's group did not
publish this finding for several years, though, because the
implications for human fertility were so troubling that the
researchers wanted to do further investigation to make sure
they were right.[2] "This chemical that we're all exposed to could
be causing an increase in miscarriages and birth defects," Dr.
Hunt recalls thinking. "I'm really worried about that."[3]

To confirm that BPA was the specific cause of the egg abnormalities, the researchers gave controlled doses of BPA to the
mice—and the same thing happened. Through a series of inves-
tigations over several years, the group determined that even a
low dose of BPA during the final stages of egg development
is enough to interfere with meiosis and cause chromosomal

abnormalities in eggs. The researchers commented that their findings had obvious relevance for chromosomal errors in human eggs because of the extraordinary similarity in chromosome processing between the two species.[4]

After Dr. Hunt's discovery, other researchers continued to study how BPA could affect fertility and soon uncovered further evidence that BPA is not only toxic to developing eggs but also interferes with the hormones that carefully coordinate the reproductive system.

In the past 15 years, study after study has shown that the small amount of BPA we are all exposed to on a daily basis could have serious health implications. The suspected toxic effects are wide-ranging and include diabetes, obesity, heart disease, and impacts on the brain and reproductive system of infants exposed during pregnancy.[5] Dr. Hunt remarked that "all of the work we've done on BPA only really increases my concern."

In 2008, one of the first large-scale studies was published showing the effects of BPA exposure on human health. Dr. Iain Lang and his colleagues analyzed data collected by the Centers for Disease Control (CDC) from over one thousand people and found a link between BPA exposure and diabetes, heart disease, and liver toxicity.[6]

These findings, which were subsequently confirmed by other large-scale studies,[7] were cause for concern because BPA is so widely used. BPA most often enters the body when people consume food and drinks that have been packaged or stored in a material that leaches BPA, but small amounts can also be absorbed through the skin from contact with products coated with BPA, such as paper receipts. By either path, BPA makes its way into the bloodstream and then into various tissues. As a result, measurable levels can be found in more than 95 percent of the US population.[8] Over 20 peer-reviewed publications have also reported measurable BPA in the bloodstream in a range of populations all over the world.[9]

While BPA causes a vast array of different biological effects, perhaps the most troubling effects involve hormonal systems. BPA has consistently been found to interfere with the activity of estrogen, testosterone, and thyroid hormones.[10] Because of this interference with endocrine systems, BPA is called an "endocrine disruptor."

It is not altogether surprising that BPA interferes with hormonal systems, because it has long been known to mimic estrogen. It was originally identified as a synthetic form of estrogen in 1936, when pharmaceutical companies were searching for a drug they could use in hormone treatment. But stronger chemicals were identified a short time later, so BPA was quickly abandoned for those purposes. Yet BPA is actually not as weak as first thought, because it disrupts the activity of several other hormones, not just estrogen.

## Are Companies Really Still Allowed to Use BPA?

In response to the large body of research on the dangers of BPA, there has been strong public pressure for regulatory agencies to take action and ban BPA. But in most jurisdictions, very little has been done. Those governments that have banned BPA have typically limited the ban to items such as baby bottles. This is a good first step because infants are likely to be particularly vulnerable to BPA, but it does not go far enough.

As Dr. Hunt exclaimed, "what the heck is this stuff doing

in consumer products, and especially products that are containers for food and beverages, if we know it's a synthetic estrogen? That really makes me mad."

In 2011, the FDA banned BPA from baby bottles and sippy cups, but in the words of the Environmental Working Group, this move was "purely cosmetic." Manufacturers had already switched to BPA-free plastic in baby bottles in response to consumer demand, and the FDA's decision was prompted by a request from a chemical industry trade association, which believed that a ban would boost consumer confidence in plastic products.[11]

Consumer demand may actually be the most powerful force we have in this battle, with the majority of reusable plastic kitchenware items in stores now claiming to be BPA free. Even the largest manufacturers of canned food have mostly phased out the use of this chemical. The real concern now is that manufacturers are simply replacing BPA with very closely related chemicals, such as bisphenol S and bisphenol F. At a practical level, this means it is much better to minimize canned food and replace plastic with glass and stainless steel, rather than simply buying products labeled as BPA free. This is important because new research indicates that BPA's cousins can compromise fertility in exactly the same way.[12]

## How Bisphenols Affect Fertility

A couple of years after Dr. Hunt's accidental experiment showing the effect of BPA on eggs from laboratory mice, evidence began to emerge that BPA significantly impairs fertility in humans too. It is now clear that women with high levels of

BPA in their system during an IVF cycle end up with fewer embryos to transfer and are less likely to become pregnant. One of the first studies hinting at this, published in 2008, showed a worrisome correlation: higher BPA levels in women who did not achieve pregnancy in IVF compared with those who did.[13] This study was troubling, but it was not until 2011 and 2012 that a body of research was published firmly establishing that anyone facing infertility should be thinking about how to limit exposure to BPA.

In 2011, a group of leading researchers and fertility specialists evaluated the link between BPA and IVF outcomes in 58 women undergoing an IVF cycle at the University of California, San Francisco Center for Reproductive Health. They found that eggs retrieved from women with higher BPA levels were less likely to fertilize.[14] This finding strongly suggests that BPA exposure reduces egg quality, which has implications not just for IVF patients but for all women trying to conceive

These harmful effects of BPA start even before the fertilization stage. Another study the same year found that BPA impacts the ovarian response to IVF stimulation medication. In that study, women with higher BPA levels had fewer eggs retrieved and lower estrogen levels.[15]

It is perhaps unsurprising then that high BPA levels may compromise IVF success rates. That was the finding of a 2012 study by researchers at the Harvard School of Public Health. In a comprehensive investigation of 174 women undergoing IVF at the Massachusetts General Hospital Fertility Center in Boston, the researchers found that women with higher BPA levels had fewer eggs retrieved, lower estrogen levels, and a lower fertilization rate.[16] The women with above-average BPA levels also had fewer five-day-old embryos available to transfer.

The same study also indicated that the impact of BPA does not end with the number of eggs and embryos formed. They also showed a link between BPA concentration in women and the failure of embryos to implant and lead to a pregnancy.[17]

The concept of implantation failure was discussed in detail in chapter 1. To review briefly, in both natural conception and IVF, only a minority of embryos are able to implant in the uterus and develop into a viable pregnancy. Implantation failure is one of the major causes of unsuccessful IVF cycles.

The Harvard researchers found that the odds of implantation failure increased with increasing levels of urinary BPA. The difference in implantation rate between women with high and low BPA levels was dramatic: The quarter of women with the highest BPA exposure had almost twice the odds of implantation failure compared to the quarter of women with the lowest BPA levels.

This study highlights a critical point—that BPA only seems to have a significant effect on the odds of success in IVF when the level of exposure is unusually high. It is typically the quarter of women with the highest levels of BPA in their systems that show poorer results in IVF. This suggests that you do not need to become vigilant about avoiding BPA entirely, but rather focus on reducing your level of exposure so you will not be in that top quarter.

There has also been another recent study finding little to no impact of BPA on IVF outcomes.[18] This outlier result led researchers at the Harvard School of Public Health and the CDC to wonder if some dietary factor could be influencing how BPA affects egg quality. In 2016 they reported a fascinating result: Consuming more than 400 micrograms of natural folate from food per day appeared to cancel out the effect of BPA.[19]

This was consistent with prior animal studies finding that folate can reduce some of the potential risks posed by BPA, but this Harvard study was key because it was looking at the precise effects of BPA on fertility in humans.

As a starting point, the researchers witnessed the same general trend as in prior studies on BPA and fertility—those women with a high level of BPA in their system before IVF had a significantly lower chance of pregnancy and live birth. Yet in the subgroup of women who consumed the most folate-rich foods, *BPA seemed to have no effect.*

Interestingly, folate from supplements did not make any difference. This could be because most supplements contain synthetic folic acid, whereas the folate present in fruits and vegetables is typically in the form of biologically active methylfolate or other forms that are readily converted to methylfolate.

It may be that only these natural forms of folate can counteract the harmful effects from BPA. Alternatively, there could be some other compound in the same foods that is actually responsible for the protective effect. Either way, the research provides reason enough to eat more folate-rich foods, particularly berries, oranges, spinach, broccoli, cauliflower, kale, asparagus, avocado, and lentils.

## BPA and Miscarriage

One reason why we still need to pay attention to minimizing BPA even with a folate-rich diet is that the chance of getting pregnant is not the only factor to consider. High levels of BPA also seem to increase the risk of miscarriage, and we do not yet know if folate is protective in that context.

One of the first studies finding a link between BPA and miscarriage was published in 2015. Forty-five women with a history of three or more first-trimester miscarriages had their BPA levels measured and compared to healthy controls. The researchers found that the average BPA level in the women with recurrent miscarriage was about three times higher than in the control group.[20] A similar trend was seen in a study in China.[21]

More recently, BPA was again implicated in raising the risk of miscarriage.[22] Researchers from Stanford University and the University of California tested BPA levels in 114 women who had recently become pregnant and who all had trouble getting pregnant or had a history of miscarriage. The researchers divided the women into four groups according to their BPA levels and were able to correlate the amount of BPA in their blood with their risk of miscarrying. Women in the top quartile of BPA were almost twice as likely to miscarry as the women in the lowest quartile.

This increased risk of miscarriage came in part from an increase in chromosomal abnormalities, which fits with what we know about BPA from the most recent animal studies. Specifically, BPA interferes with chromosome processing in developing eggs.[23] But women with higher BPA levels were also more likely to miscarry even where the fetus was chromosomally normal. Additional research published in 2016 suggests this could be the result of interfering with progesterone signaling, thereby making the uterine lining less receptive in early pregnancy.[24]

Again, however, it is important to keep in mind that it is

higher levels of BPA associated with miscarriage risk. In the study described above, the increase in miscarriage rate was only statistically significant in the quarter of women with the highest BPA level. To both improve your odds of conceiving and prevent miscarriage, the main goal is simply to get out of that top quarter; to lower your overall exposure rather than avoid all possible sources of BPA.

## How to Avoid BPA without Becoming Paranoid

The good news about BPA is that there is a lot you can do to reduce your exposure, and once you take a few simple steps, the amount of BPA in your system will decrease rapidly.[25] The most important time for reducing your exposure to BPA is in the three or four months before you try to conceive, but it is never too early or too late to start.

So where exactly should you begin? The first step I recommend is to look for plastic items in your kitchen that you can easily replace with glass or stainless steel. The highest priority should be items that are quite old or come into contact with hot food or drinks. Typically, these are the top items to replace:

- Reusable food storage containers

- Microwave-safe bowls

- Reusable plastic water bottles and cups

- Plastic tea kettles

- Colanders

- Blender containers that have been used with hot soups

For these items, glass and stainless steel are the best choice, despite the fact that many newer plastic kitchenware items are labeled as BPA free. As mentioned earlier, many manufacturers have simply replaced BPA with closely related compounds, such as bisphenol S (BPS). These chemicals may be just as much of a concern, with recent studies finding that BPS can contribute to chromosomal errors in eggs in just the same way as BPA.[26]

The plastic most likely to contain compounds closely related to BPA is polycarbonate, which is used to make hard, reusable plastic and is often marked as "PC" or with the number 7 in the recycling symbol. Safer types of plastic include polypropylene ("PP" or number 5) or high-density polyethylene (HDPE or number 2). These plastics may still leach hormone-disrupting chemicals under certain circumstances,[27] but the risk is relatively low if they are treated carefully.

When it comes to chemicals leaching from plastic, the main risk factors are heat, acid, UV light, and contact with liquids. It probably goes without saying that you should not drink coffee from a reusable plastic travel mug or blend hot soups in a blender made from plastic. A coffee machine with plastic internal parts may also be problematic and should ideally be replaced with a glass or stainless steel French press. On the other hand, you can be less concerned about containers that are used to store dry goods, such as rice and flour, because any chemicals present are much less likely to transfer.

When it comes to water filters and bottled water, the answer is less clear. Reusable plastic water bottles are made of a type of plastic that should not contain BPA, but if the water has been in the bottle for months or years, under unknown storage conditions, there is the possibility of some degree of contamination from other chemicals, such as phthalates (discussed in the next chapter). For this reason, it is preferable to drink plastic bottled water only when you have no other practical option. The best choice is filtered tap water (with a reusable stainless steel water bottle), or water bottled in glass.

Finding an affordable water filter without plastic is often quite difficult, so this is one situation where compromise is likely needed for the sake of practicality. Even though most water filters contain some plastic components, there is no heat involved and the water is typically only in contact with the plastic for short periods of time, particularly in the case of faucet, refrigerator, or under-counter filters. If you use a plastic filter pitcher jug, the water may sit in the plastic for longer periods of time, so it is important to treat the plastic carefully and replace it once it becomes scratched, or if it has been washed in the dishwasher.

See **www.itstartswiththeegg.com/purging-plastics** for further advice on prioritizing what to replace and my recommended water filters and other kitchenware products.

Many people who begin casting a suspicious eye over the plastic in their kitchen inevitably wonder if all the plastic packaging on their food is troubling too. Most of the time, the answer is no. While it pays to make some slightly different choices at the supermarket, plastic food packaging is not the main enemy. Rather, it is more helpful to avoid highly processed ingredients in favor of whole foods closer to their natural state. That is because food is most likely to contain a significant amount of BPA or similar chemicals if it has been highly processed, canned, or prepared outside the home.

These foods are higher in BPA because factories and restaurants make extensive use of plastic containers and processing equipment, and it is often washed with scalding hot water. By limiting highly processed junk foods and eating more food made in the home from whole, unprocessed ingredients, you can dramatically lower your level of BPA exposure, even if you are still eating foods that are packaged in plastic.[28]

Historically, canned food has been one of the highest sources of BPA exposure, although the situation is now in a state of flux. Most major manufacturers have switched to BPA-free can linings, but they are free to use a range of replacements. Some are benign; some are likely just as bad or worse than BPA. Unfortunately, there is typically no way to know what has been used for any given product. We do know that canned tomatoes are the most important food to avoid, because the acidity increases the leaching of chemicals from the can lining.[29] Canned beans are less problematic, but it is still preferable to use dried or frozen beans when you can.

One other possible source of BPA at the supermarket is the paper receipt you are handed. The thermal paper used for receipts can be coated with BPA or other closely related chemicals.[30] After several hours, a small amount can be absorbed through the skin.[31] Retail employees who touch receipts throughout their workday can therefore have very high levels of BPA in their systems.[32] Occasionally handling receipts while shopping is likely not something to worry about excessively, but it is best to wash your hands when you return home.

The bottom line is that starting to minimize your exposure to BPA can be daunting, but it is worth the trouble given the likely impact on your reproductive health. Instead of worrying about BPA on a daily basis, the best approach is to make a few high-priority changes that make the most difference. It is also important to remember that there is no need to become obsessed with removing BPA from your life; the goal is simply to remove the worst offenders to reduce your overall level of exposure.

## Reader story: Anna Rapp

After two years of trying to get pregnant, with multiple early miscarriages, endometriosis, an MTHFR mutation, low AMH, low antral follicle count, and an FSH reading of 34, I was told that I would never have a baby with my own eggs—at the age of 32. I was frustrated, sad, and on the verge of depression. I was given one shot at IVF, but only if I lowered my FSH significantly.

After reading *It Starts with the Egg*, I embarked on a program of lifestyle changes, with a particular focus on a nourishing diet, a daily mind-body practice, and reducing toxins. I replaced as much plastic in the kitchen as possible, threw away fragranced cleaning and beauty products, and stopped eating canned food. I also stopped using nail polish and started buying more organic food. All this work, together with my fertility-friendly diet and other strategies, lowered my FSH to 12 and helped me get happy and healthy while preparing for IVF. I never did try IVF—I was pregnant naturally in less than three months!

Read more from Anna on her blog, To Make a Mommy

## BPA Exposure During Pregnancy

Interestingly, the payoff for avoiding BPA does not end when you become pregnant—it is also beneficial for the health of your baby. Researchers have long suspected that a developing fetus is particularly vulnerable to the toxic effects of BPA.[33] It has been shown that BPA crosses the placenta from the mother's bloodstream into the baby, and BPA has been found in both the amniotic fluid and the fetus during pregnancy.[34]

A large number of studies have suggested a link between exposure to BPA during pregnancy and a variety of long-term health consequences, particularly for brain development and the reproductive system.[35] In one such study, prenatal exposure was associated with behavioral abnormalities in young children.[36] While it still is not known exactly what risks BPA poses during pregnancy, setting up a healthier kitchen and getting in the habit of limiting your exposure has a dual advantage of both protecting your fertility and protecting your baby when you do become pregnant.

## Action Steps
### Basic, Intermediate, and Advanced Plans

- It is never too early or too late to start reducing your exposure to BPA.

- Reduce your exposure by

> › replacing any plastic kitchenware that comes into contact with hot food or drinks.

> › using a stainless steel water bottle.

> › minimizing canned and highly processed foods.

> › preparing more meals at home, using whole, natural ingredients.

> › taking care when using plastic (even if it says "BPA free") by choosing polypropylene or HDPE plastic and washing by hand.

> › washing your hands when you return home after handling paper receipts.

- It is also important to continue these steps for limiting your exposure to BPA when you become pregnant, to protect your growing baby.

# CHAPTER 3

# Phthalates and Other Toxins

*"Big, sweeping life changes really boil down to small, everyday decisions."*

—ALI VINCENT

BPA IS UNFORTUNATELY just one example of how chemicals that act as endocrine disruptors can stand in the way of your ability to get pregnant. Another type of toxin that may impair egg quality and fertility is a group of chemicals known as phthalates (pronounced THAL-lates).

Phthalates are widely used in plastic, vinyl, cleaning products, nail polish, and fragrances.[1] Just like BPA, these chemicals can compromise the activity of hormones that are critical for fertility.[2] By avoiding a small number of "worst offenders" that contribute most to daily phthalate exposure, you can quickly reduce the level of these chemicals in your body, creating a safer environment for your developing eggs and your future pregnancy.

## The Current State of Play on Phthalates

For decades, scientists have known that phthalates can alter the levels and activity of hormones in the body. Phthalates are now officially recognized as a reproductive toxin in the European Union,[3] and the U.S. FDA has also acknowledged that phthalates are endocrine disruptors.[4]

As a result of these known toxic effects, certain phthalates have been banned in children's toys in Europe since 1999, and in the United States since 2008. Similar bans are also in place in Canada and Australia. As the European Commission said in 1999, the ban was intended "to protect the youngest and most vulnerable amongst us. We received scientific advice that phthalates pose a serious risk to human health."[5]

Yet if phthalates pose a serious risk to human health, why has no action been taken to ban phthalates more widely? If it is beyond question that phthalates are toxic to babies and young children, why is little attention paid to the potential toxic effects before and during pregnancy?

In the words of a leading researcher in the field, Dr. Shanna Swan: "eliminating these phthalates from children's toys—I think it is important...—but I would not do that at the expense of eliminating phthalates in products to which pregnant women are exposed. Because that is the most critical target for phthalates."[6]

Clearly any regulation that does exist is not working, because biologically active forms of phthalates have been detected in 95 percent of pregnant women.[7] This finding is not all that surprising given that phthalates are widely used in everything from fabric softeners to food processing equipment to perfumes. As a result, these chemicals can be found in the bloodstream of the vast majority of people tested in the United States, Europe, and Asia.[8]

The fact that almost all women are exposed to phthalates during pregnancy is troubling because there is strong evidence that high levels of these chemicals can negatively impact a developing fetus. This is reason enough to start to remove phthalates from your home now in order to protect your growing baby when you do become pregnant. But the sooner you start, the better, because evidence is also emerging that high levels of phthalates may contribute to poor egg quality and therefore infertility.

## Phthalates and Fertility

There are still many unknowns when it comes to the precise impact of phthalates on fertility. Yet what little evidence we do have is very troubling, at least for high levels of exposure.

The first evidence to emerge showed that high doses of phthalates interfered with fertility in laboratory animals. In one of the earliest studies, rats given high doses of a particular phthalate simply stopped ovulating.[9] The phthalate used in this study, called DEHP, is the type most commonly found in processed food, so this discovery was quite disturbing.

Gradually the initial findings on the impact of high doses in animals were extended to show that various different phthalates have damaging effects on the human reproductive system too.[10]

Many of the early human studies focused on male fertility, with research finding that phthalate exposure significantly affects sperm quality.[11] These chemicals seem to damage sperm in a variety of ways, including altering hormone levels and causing oxidative stress.[12] Both of these mechanisms would suggest that female fertility could be similarly affected. The latest research has indeed found that phthalates harm developing eggs in much the same way.

## What Happens to Eggs Exposed to Phthalates?

For the past decade, researchers have been demonstrating in animal and laboratory studies that phthalates compromise egg development.[13] This appears to occur in part because these chemicals decrease production of estrogen, which is one of the main drivers of egg development.[14]

But the effect of phthalates does not end with compromising the ability of eggs to mature properly. The next critical step before pregnancy—embryo survival—could also be disturbed. This is a stage of conception you have probably not given much thought to unless you have been through an IVF cycle in which your fertilized embryos did not make it to the five-day mark. Unfortunately, this is not uncommon, and in a typical IVF cycle, many embryos do not survive those first few days before they are transferred to the uterus. Embryo survival is also critical when trying to conceive naturally.

One of the ways phthalates likely compromise egg and embryo quality is by causing oxidative stress.[15] Oxidative stress occurs when a cell produces more reactive oxygen molecules (commonly known as free radicals or oxidants) than it can handle. Antioxidants within the cell normally keep these reactive molecules in check, but if they cannot keep up, reactive molecules can damage the cell. This state is called oxidative stress.

Oxidative stress causes ovarian follicles to die off[16] and has been linked to the age-related decline in fertility, endometriosis, and unexplained infertility.[17] Studies have shown that exposure to phthalates may be one contributing factor to oxidative stress in developing eggs and therefore contribute to infertility.

In the largest human study on phthalates and oxidative stress, looking at data from approximately 10,000 people in the United States collected over eight years, people with higher levels of several phthalates had higher levels of inflammation and oxidative stress.[18]

This type of large population study can only establish a link, not a cause-and-effect relationship. But that is where animal and laboratory studies are useful because they show at a molecular level that phthalates do cause oxidative stress in a variety of cells, including eggs. This happens because phthalates block our natural antioxidant enzymes, which would otherwise protect cells from damage by free radicals.

Early studies found that a particular phthalate, DEHP, alters the activity of key antioxidant enzymes in the liver and in the cells that produce sperm, resulting in oxidative stress.[19] In 2011, this was also shown to happen in developing eggs too.[20] In other words, phthalates weaken eggs' natural antioxidant defense systems.

The implication from all these studies—that phthalates could impact IVF outcomes—was finally confirmed in 2016. In a study by Harvard researchers involving 250 women undergoing IVF, it was found that the women with higher levels of DEHP had fewer eggs retrieved and were significantly less likely to become pregnant. When compared to women with the lowest phthalate levels, those with the highest levels were 20 percent less likely to give birth.[21]

In addition, phthalate exposure has been associated with an increased risk of endometriosis.[22] Endometriosis is a poorly understood condition in which cells from the lining of the uterus find their way to other places in the pelvis, causing pain and impaired fertility.

Even though it is not yet known what causes endometriosis, researchers suspect that phthalate exposure could be one of many contributing factors. This is because the vast majority of studies examining this issue have shown significantly higher levels of phthalates in women with endometriosis than those without the condition.[23] In one of the largest studies to date, researchers at the National Institutes of Health, the University of Utah, and several other institutions analyzed phthalate levels in over four hundred women.[24] They found a higher level of six different phthalate compounds in women with endometriosis. In this study, higher phthalate levels were in fact associated with a twofold increase in the rate of endometriosis.

This by no means suggests that reducing your exposure to phthalates will improve or prevent endometriosis; we simply do not know enough to conclude that. But the research on a possible connection between phthalates and endometriosis serves as a warning that phthalates could be impacting our reproductive systems in ways that are not yet understood.

## Miscarriage

In addition to making it more difficult to become pregnant, women with high levels of phthalates in their system before they conceive may be more likely to miscarry.[25] This link was first reported by researchers in Denmark, who followed a group of women trying to get pregnant over six months. The researchers tested the women for a range of phthalates and also tested for the pregnancy hormone HCG at specific times each month. Because of this regular testing for HCG, even very early pregnancy losses were detected, including those that occurred before the women even knew they were pregnant. The researchers found that a higher level of one particular phthalate before pregnancy was linked to a higher rate of miscarriage in general, but especially very early losses.

In a 2016 study, researchers at Harvard Medical School and the prestigious Massachusetts General Hospital looked at this question further, by measuring phthalate levels in 250 women who conceived by IVF. The researchers again found that the quarter of women with the highest phthalate levels had a significantly higher risk of miscarriage. The difference was especially marked for so-called "biochemical" pregnancies, which are very early miscarriages that occur before the fetus is visible on ultrasound, typically at around six weeks.

The link between miscarriage and toxins in our homes may be disheartening, but it is actually very good news, because it means there is one more risk factor we can change, simply by making smarter choices. The studies also indicate that it is the very high levels we need to be most concerned about. The goal is therefore not to avoid phthalates completely (which would be impossible), but rather to make sure you are not one of the minority of women with unusually high levels.

## Reducing Your Exposure to Phthalates

Phthalates are found in a variety of different places—from cosmetics to laundry products to food. Their widespread use makes it difficult to know where to begin, but the latest studies provide useful information to guide decisions on the types of phthalates that matter most, and how to make the most difference to your overall level of exposure.

As a starting point, in the major studies to date linking phthalates to miscarriage, the specific type of phthalate implicated is one that leaches from vinyl/PVC plastic (this phthalate is known as DEHP. In the body it is broken down into a variety of other compounds, such as MEHP).

Although PVC is found in many different places, new research indicates that the major way that DEHP gets into our bodies is actually through food.[26] In particular, fast food and highly processed food.

In one of the largest studies on this issue, involving almost nine thousand people, researchers measured phthalate levels and compared the results against the participant's consumption of fast food over a 24-hour period.[27] They found that people who ate at least one fast-food meal had much higher phthalate levels. Specifically, they had a 24 percent higher level of DEHP, the particular phthalate linked to miscarriage.

This study suggests that simply making more meals at home is one of the most powerful ways to minimize exposure to the phthalate of greatest concern. Other research further confirms that preparing and storing meals without plastic, using fresh ingredients, can dramatically lower phthalate levels in just a few days.

That was found in a study of five families in San Francisco, where participants had meals prepared for them from organic and unprocessed ingredients. The meals were made and stored without plastic utensils or containers, and the participants were only allowed to drink coffee made in a French press rather than a coffee machine with plastic parts. After only a couple of days, the levels of many phthalates fell by over 50 percent.[28]

This study also tried to reduce the use of ingredients that were packaged in plastic, but we know from further studies that the final packaging of most unprocessed, natural ingredients is not the major concern. As one example, researchers in Canada recently measured phthalates in over 100 samples of meat (beef, pork, and chicken), fish, and cheese, packaged mostly in cling films. Phthalates were not detected in the packaging.[29] The only food with measurable phthalate levels was cheese (likely from processing) and even then the level was relatively low.

Additional studies have also found that packaging makes a relatively small contribution to the total amount of phthalates in food. In an investigation into a variety of processed and unprocessed foods, another study concluded that "processing—and not packaging—was the most important contamination source."[30] This makes a lot of sense, given that the manufacturing process often uses plastic containers and equipment, much of which is likely sterilized with scalding hot water.

That is not to say that food packaging is completely in the clear. Although the main sources of phthalates are fast food and highly processed foods, there are a couple of circumstances in which it may make sense to avoid plastic when you can.

Researchers have found, for example, that milk has much

lower phthalate levels when packaged in glass than plastic.[31] As a more general principle, for phthalates to leach from the container into food, the main risk factors are heat, acid, or liquid. As a result, it is preferable to buy milk, oil, drinks, and condiments in glass bottles or other alternatives to plastic when possible. It is also advisable to buy water in plastic bottles only when necessary, because researchers have consistently found that water packaged in these plastic bottles contains much higher phthalate levels than water packaged in glass bottles.[32] It probably also goes without saying that you should also avoid any hot foods in plastic containers.

For the most part, however, you should feel comfortable buying food in plastic containers or bags, as long as you are placing more emphasis on natural ingredients such as nuts, legumes, unprocessed grains, meat, eggs, fish, fruit, and vegetables. The more these foods contribute to your overall diet, and the more you prepare meals yourself at home, the lower your levels of the phthalate that matters most.

## Prioritizing the Strategies for Other Phthalates

To take phthalate-avoidance to the next level and start minimizing your exposure to other phthalates that do not necessarily contribute to miscarriage risk but may still compromise fertility in other ways, the next place to look is your bathroom. The major way we are exposed to other phthalates is from products such as hairspray, perfume, and nail polish, along with air fresheners and fabric softeners.[33] The phthalates in these products can be readily absorbed through the skin or inhaled from the air.[34]

Although phthalates can be found in just about anything fragranced, and there is advantage to eventually moving toward a fragrance-free home, the best place to start is with the worst offenders: nail polish, perfume, and hairspray. All three of these products often contain high concentrations of phthalates as a structural part of the product.

Nail polish typically has a higher concentration of phthalates than any other cosmetic product and the safest option is to stop wearing nail polish while trying to conceive.[35] Nail polish may also contain other nasty chemicals such as formaldehyde and toluene, both of which have been linked to reduced fertility and increased risk of miscarriage.[36] Many different studies across the world have concluded that women exposed to formaldehyde on a daily basis through their workplace (nail salons, hospitals, and laboratories) have more than twice the chance of miscarriage.[37]

Many nail polish brands now claim to be phthalate free and formaldehyde free, however these claims must be treated with some skepticism. Studies have found that labeling of nail polish is often very inaccurate, with many brands containing high levels of phthalates despite claims to the contrary.

Buying nail polish labeled as "phthalate free" is still a safer option than traditional formulations, but in the end we may not be able to trust what manufacturers say. The best brands are probably those sold at WholeFoods or ranked as less toxic by the Environmental Working Group's Skin Deep Cosmetics Database.

The next "worst offender" when it comes to phthalates is perfume.[38] Studies have found that women who wear perfume can have double the concentration of some phthalates in their system. Perfumes are also a cocktail of dozens of other chemicals that can potentially cause allergies and disrupt hormones, many of which have never been tested for safety. If you cannot give up fragrance altogether, consider switching to all-natural fragrances or body lotions scented with natural essential oils and labeled as "phthalate free."

Although perfume contains an unusually high concentration, small amounts of phthalates may also be added to virtually anything fragranced, including skin care, hair care, air fresheners, cleaning sprays, laundry detergent, and fabric softener. Companies are allowed to do this because of a loophole whereby manufacturers are not required to identify individual ingredients in fragrances. Anytime you see the word "fragrance" in a list of ingredients, phthalates may be present.

The best solution is to start switching to fragrance-free products to the extent your budget allows. That does not mean you have to immediately throw away every single fragranced item in your home, but to replace what you can when you can. With skin care products, the highest priority item is probably your body lotion. Since it is applied over a larger surface area of skin, the chemicals have more opportunity to be absorbed. Fabric softener is another top item to either replace or stop using altogether, because it can have quite high concentrations of phthalates. Natural wool dryer balls are a good alternative.

How much further you choose to go in replacing your cosmetics and cleaning products is up to you, but every little bit helps. Additional items to consider replacing include PVC shower curtains and yoga mats. Look for a shower curtain made from nylon, cotton, or polyester, and a yoga mat labeled "PVC free" or "phthalate free."

> For up to date recommendations on phthalate-free skin care, hair care, cleaning, and laundry products, visit **www.itstartswiththeegg.com/product-guide**

At the end of the day, it is up to you to decide which changes are easiest for you to make and how careful you want to be. Replacing skin care products with brands that emphasize natural ingredients has the added bonus of not only reducing your exposure to phthalates but also a host of other potentially toxic chemicals, such as parabens.

In one recent study, Harvard researchers suggested that propyl-paraben, a common preservative in personal care products, is linked to diminished ovarian reserve.[39] Cosmetics companies that go to the trouble of eliminating phthalates from their products are more likely to stay away from these other harmful chemicals too.

Starting the process of reducing phthalates in your home will also have even greater benefits once you do become pregnant. That is because minimizing your exposure throughout pregnancy may also help reduce your risk of premature birth and the risk of rare reproductive abnormalities in baby boys.[40] Avoiding phthalates will also support your baby's brain development, with lower levels during pregnancy linked to better language development in children.[41]

## The Bigger Picture

If you feel inspired to do even more to create a nontoxic home, there are of course other steps you can take. The world is also full of many other synthetic chemicals, but in general we know very little about how they affect fertility.

If you want to be particularly cautious and minimize exposure to other known hormone disruptors, the best place to start is the Environmental Working Group's Dirty Dozen list of endocrine disruptors.[42] In addition to BPA and phthalates, this list contains ten other common toxins that you can avoid in surprisingly simple ways:

**Dioxin**: Choose low-fat meat and dairy, and use olive oil instead of butter.

**Atrazine**: Buy more organic fruit and vegetables, and use a water filter certified to remove atrazine (see the Environmental Working Group's Water Filter Buying Guide[43]).

**Perchlorate**: Although difficult to avoid, you can minimize its potential to disrupt thyroid hormones by getting enough iodine in your diet, such as through iodized salt.

**Fire Retardants**: These chemicals have recently been linked to a higher risk of miscarriage.[44] Flame retardants are released into household dust from furniture, rugs, and electronics. The best way to minimize exposure is regularly vacuuming and dusting with a damp cloth.

**Lead**: Buy a water filter certified to remove lead, and take off your shoes at the door.

**Arsenic**: Use a water filter certified to remove arsenic.

**Mercury**: Choose low-mercury fish, and don't handle the

new compact-fluorescent light bulbs. If dropped and broken, these bulbs release mercury vapors into the air.

**Perfluorinated Chemicals** (PFCs): Use stainless steel and cast iron cookware instead of nonstick pans. Newer nonstick pans that are labeled as free of "PFOA" and "PTFE" are a much better alternative to conventional Teflon.

**Organophosphate Pesticides**: Buy organic fruit and vegetables if you can, or choose varieties less likely to be contaminated with high levels of pesticides—typically those with a protective outer peel such as pineapple, mango, kiwi, corn, peas, onion, cabbage, and avocado.

**Glycol Ethers**: Avoid cleaning products containing 2-butoxyethanol (EGBE) and methoxydiglycol (DEGME).

To this list we should add quaternary ammonium compounds, which appear to compromise fertility and increase the risk of birth defects, at least in initial animal studies.[45] This family of chemicals is used in many common disinfectant sprays and wipes, along with alcohol-free hand sanitizers (often appearing on the label as benzalkonium chloride). Alcohol and vinegar are much safer alternatives.

While the risk of harm from quaternary ammonium compounds is still under investigation, the research in this area further emphasizes the value in choosing natural, nontoxic household products rather than gambling with the dozens of untested chemicals found in conventional brands.

As Dr. Swan explained, "I think we have now a lot of data that environmental chemicals can and do lower sperm count, impact time to conception, increase fetal loss in early pregnancy, and affect pregnancy outcomes. Do we need more studies? Of course we do. But do we have enough information to act on these studies that we have? I say that we do."[46]

Fortunately, manufacturers are responding to the growing consumer demand for more natural and nontoxic products, and it is easier than ever to find safer products. In this regard, two helpful tools are the Environmental Working Group's Skin Deep Database and the ThinkDirty app, both of which rate the ingredients of hundreds of thousands of products to help you find safer options.

## Action Steps
### *Basic, Intermediate,* and *Advanced Plans*

- Reduce phthalate exposure from food by preparing more meals at home, using minimally processed ingredients.

- Try to avoid using conventional perfume, hair spray, nail polish, and fabric softener.

- To the extent your budget permits, start replacing other hair care and skin care products with ones labeled fragrance free or, better yet, phthalate free.

- When buying cleaning and laundry products, look for brands that are plant based, fragrance free, or phthalate free.

- For detailed product recommendations, see www.itstartswiththeegg.com/product-guide.

# CHAPTER 4

# Unexpected
# Obstacles to Fertility

*"Discovery consists of seeing what everybody has
seen and thinking what nobody has thought."*
—ALBERT SZENT-GYORGYI

I F YOU ARE having trouble conceiving or have had one or more miscarriages, you should ask your doctor to test you for several easily treated conditions that are often missed: vitamin D deficiency, underactive thyroid, and celiac disease. Not all doctors will think about testing for these conditions unless you ask, but each condition has a surprisingly strong link to infertility and miscarriage. Any one of these factors could be the missing link in your treatment plan and, once corrected, will give you the best chance of a healthy pregnancy.

## Surprising Factor 1: Vitamin D

In the past decade, vitamin D has become a hot area of research. Low levels of vitamin D have now been implicated in a wide variety of diseases, including diabetes, cancer, obesity, multiple sclerosis, and arthritis. Although the research on the role of vitamin D and fertility has only just begun and is somewhat inconsistent, several studies indicate that low levels of vitamin D may negatively impact fertility.[1]

In one of the most compelling studies, which was published in 2012, researchers at Columbia University and the University of Southern California (USC) measured vitamin D levels in nearly two hundred women undergoing IVF. Of the Caucasian women in the group, the odds of pregnancy were *four times* higher for women with high vitamin D levels compared to those with a vitamin D deficiency.[2]

An earlier study also found that in the group of women with the highest vitamin D levels, 47 percent became pregnant, while among women with low vitamin D levels, the pregnancy rate was only 20 percent.[3] Another more recent IVF study revealed a higher fertilization and implantation rate in a group of women with higher vitamin D levels.[4]

It is not yet known how vitamin D is involved in fertility, but researchers suspect that one role is making the uterine lining more receptive to pregnancy.[5] There are specific receptors for vitamin D in cells in the ovaries and the uterus.[6] Vitamin D also plays a role in hormone production. A deficiency may contribute to infertility by interrupting the estrogen system and also reducing production of antimullerian hormone (AMH), which is involved in the growth of ovarian follicles.[7] In addition, low vitamin D levels appear to contribute to endometriosis and PCOS.[8]

## Vitamin D and miscarriage

Vitamin D is also particularly important for preventing miscarriage. That was the finding of several clinical studies published in 2018, which reported that women who had adequate vitamin D levels before they became pregnant had a significantly lower risk of miscarriage.[9] In one of the studies, conducted by the National Institutes of Health, women who had sufficient preconception vitamin D levels were 10 percent more likely to become pregnant and 15 percent more likely to give birth, compared to those with insufficient levels. In this study, the cut-off value characterized as "sufficient" was 30 nanograms per milliliter (ng/ml), yet the preferred level is likely higher. Each 10 ng/ml increase in preconception vitamin D was associated with a 12 percent lower risk of pregnancy loss.

Separate research has also shown a clear link between vitamin D levels and the immune factors often involved in recurrent miscarriage, such as natural killer cells and markers of systemic inflammation.[10] Women with higher vitamin D levels are less likely to have these immune abnormalities. This suggests that supplementing with vitamin D could be particularly helpful if you have a history of miscarriage caused by immune factors.

## Optimal vitamin D levels

Vitamin D deficiencies are surprisingly common, particularly in cooler climates. By some estimates, as much as 36 percent of the United States population is deficient, even with the most conservative cut-off value.[11] There is actually a great deal of controversy over exactly what level of vitamin D counts as a deficiency. Conventionally, 20 ng/ml has been the minimum recommended level, but that is based on preserving bone health.

As mentioned above, the recent miscarriage studies indicate that 30 ng/ml (75 nmol/l) should be considered the bare minimum. Up to 80 percent of women have vitamin D levels below this point.[12] New research has found that an even higher level is preferred to balance the immune system and allow optimal development of the placenta.[13] As discussed in detail in my upcoming pregnancy book (www.itstartswiththeegg.com/sequel), the latest studies show that the optimal vitamin D level is likely at least 40 ng/mL (100 nmol/L).

### Vitamin D Cut-off Levels for Fertility and Miscarriage Prevention

- Deficient: below 20 ng/ml (50 nmol/l)
- Insufficient: 20–30 ng/ml (50–75 nmol/l)
- Sufficient: at least 30 ngl/ml (75 nmol/l)
- Optimal: at least 40 ng/mL (100 nmol/L)

### Supplementing with vitamin D

Unless you live in a tropical climate and get significant daily sun exposure, it is highly likely that your vitamin D level is too low and you will need to supplement. The necessary dose depends on just how deficient you are and how high you are aiming, so it is best to have your level tested and seek your doctor's advice on the appropriate dose. If your doctor is reluctant to run the test, it is likely best to assume you have a mild deficiency and supplement accordingly.

The Endocrine Society recommends that all adults who are vitamin D deficient should be treated with 6000–10000 IU of vitamin D per day in the short term (typically two weeks), followed by a lower ongoing maintenance dose. The standard maintenance dose is typically 2000 IU, yet that is aimed at maintaining "normal" levels, not the higher levels that are optimal for fertility and pregnancy.

Studies indicate that many women need approximately 4000 IU per day to maintain vitamin D levels above 40 ng/mL (100 nmol/L). Yet there are wide variations in how much vitamin D any given person needs to reach and maintain the optimal level, depending on genetics and sun exposure. If your current level is already between 30 and 40 ng/mL, you may only need to add an additional 2000 IU per day. On the other hand, it is possible that you may require a higher dose, such as 5000 IU per day.

Erring on the side of a higher dose could be helpful if you have any condition associated with inflammation or autoimmunity, such as thyroid disease, endometriosis, or a history of recurrent miscarriage. Dr. Amy Myers, physician and author of *The Autoimmune Solution*, recommends a target level of 60–90 ng/mL for those with thyroid conditions or other autoimmune diseases. To reach this level, consider supplementing with 10,000 IU per day for two weeks, then 5000 IU per day as a maintenance dosage, with repeat blood testing to confirm that you have reached the optimal range.

The main concern with taking too much vitamin D is raising blood calcium levels, since vitamin D improves calcium absorption from food. Yet the Mayo Clinic advises that this problem has been reported with 60,000 IU per day for several months. In a study of patients with multiple sclerosis, 20,000 IU per day for 12 weeks reduced inflammatory immune cells without causing a significant rise in calcium levels.[14]

Based on this study and other current evidence, it appears that high blood calcium levels are unlikely at just 5000 IU per day. Even so, it may still be prudent to lower your dairy intake and occasionally check your blood calcium levels if you are taking this dose long-term.

In addition, those taking higher doses of vitamin D for long periods of time are often also advised to add a vitamin K2 supplement. This is intended to direct any excess calcium into strengthening bones, rather than forming calcium deposits in blood vessels. If you choose to add a K2 supplement, it may be best to keep the dose relatively low, such as 45 micrograms, because supplementing with vitamin K2 appears to reduce testosterone.[15] This is helpful for those with PCOS, but not for those with diminished ovarian reserve.

To obtain the most benefit from a vitamin D supplement, it is best to choose vitamin D3 formulated in oil-based drops or an oil-based soft gel capsule, rather than a solid tablet, and to take it with a meal containing some fat. These measures significantly improve the absorption of vitamin D because it is a fat-soluble vitamin.[16] (For recommended brands, see www.itstartswiththeegg.com/supplements.)

### Surprising Factor 2: Hypothyroidism

If you have been struggling with infertility or miscarriages, you should also ask your doctor to check your thyroid hormone and antibody levels. Even very mild thyroid conditions can dramatically increase the risk of miscarriage. In addition, hypothyroidism (underactive thyroid) is common in women with premature ovarian failure, unexplained infertility, and ovulation disorders.

The link between miscarriage and thyroid disorders was discovered by accident more than 20 years ago. The research project that uncovered the link was originally designed to understand why some women develop thyroid disorders after they give birth. To investigate this, more than five hundred women in New York were screened for thyroid hormones and thyroid antibodies in the first trimester of pregnancy. Thyroid antibodies were tested because their presence is a sign that the immune system is mounting an attack on the thyroid, which is the most common cause of hypothyroidism.[17]

As this study unfolded, the researchers noticed a high number of miscarriages in the women who tested positive for thyroid antibodies. The researchers decided to look at the miscarriage rates more closely and found that in women with thyroid antibodies, the miscarriage rate more than doubled.[18] This finding was so unexpected that the researchers were not sure whether the results showed a real link or just reflected a statistical fluke.[19]

In the 20 years since that initial research, dozens of studies have confirmed that having an autoimmune thyroid disorder significantly increases the risk of miscarriage. In a large study in Pakistan published in 2006, the miscarriage rate was even higher than earlier studies suggested—36 percent in women who tested thyroid antibody positive compared to just 1.8 percent for those without thyroid antibodies.[20]

Thyroid conditions are also extremely common in women with recurrent miscarriage—typically defined as women who have lost three or more pregnancies. Thyroid antibodies are present in more than a third of women with recurrent miscarriage, compared to 7–13 percent of women without a history of miscarriage.[21]

Doctors are not entirely sure why thyroid antibodies pose such a problem in early pregnancy. One of the most puzzling facts is that having antibodies against the thyroid increases the miscarriage risk significantly, even when the thyroid is still functioning well and thyroid hormone levels are basically normal.[22] In these cases, researchers believe thyroid antibodies may contribute to miscarriage risk by reducing the ability of the thyroid to rise to the demand of making extra hormones during pregnancy. That is, even when the thyroid is functioning normally before pregnancy, thyroid autoimmunity may result in a small decrease in the ability of the thyroid to function, which can be very detrimental in early pregnancy.

Even though thyroid antibodies do raise miscarriage rates in women without any obvious decline in thyroid function, the miscarriage rate is especially high when tests show that in addition to thyroid antibodies, the hormone levels are abnormal because the thyroid is struggling to keep up.[23] Researchers have found that the miscarriage rate is 69 percent higher in women with a clearly underactive thyroid gland and hormonal imbalances.[24]

This, believe it or not, is good news because a firm link between the disruption of thyroid hormones and miscarriage implies that correcting thyroid hormone levels may also help prevent miscarriage. Just as we would hope, initial research shows that thyroid hormone treatment is incredibly effective at reducing miscarriage rates.

For example, a study in Italy of women with untreated thyroid antibodies found a miscarriage rate of 13.8 percent compared to 2.4 percent in women without thyroid problems. But when women with thyroid antibodies received thyroid hormone treatments during pregnancy, the miscarriage rate dropped to just 3.5 percent—much lower than untreated women and approaching that of women without any thyroid problems.[25] These positive results have been seen in several other studies,[26] providing powerful evidence that treating hypothyroidism can make a significant difference to miscarriage rates.

Thyroid disorders are, however, not just related to miscarriage—they are also very common in women with unexplained infertility, ovulation disorders, and premature ovarian failure.

Premature ovarian failure is a condition in which the number and quality of eggs severely limits fertility. IVF is often the only path to becoming pregnant in women with this diagnosis, and even then the success rates are very low. Cycles are often canceled because not enough eggs grow and mature in response to stimulation medication. Premature ovarian failure is poorly understood, but one factor that has recently emerged is the link to thyroid disorders.

It has become apparent that even a very mild reduction in thyroid activity, a condition called "subclinical" hypothyroidism, could be a major contributor to premature ovarian failure. In recent studies, while only 4 percent of healthy women were found to have subclinical hypothyroidism, the rate increased to 15 percent of women with ovulatory infertility and 40 percent of women with premature ovarian failure.[27]

Another study demonstrated that 20 percent of women with ovulation disorders have subclinical hypothyroidism, finding that this condition is more than twice as common in women with ovulation disorders as in women with normal ovulation (20.5 percent versus 8.3 percent).[28]

As with miscarriage rates, the results of treatment with thyroid hormones are very encouraging. In one such study, after infertile women with subclinical hypothyroidism were treated with the synthetic thyroid hormone levothyroxine, 44 percent of the women became pregnant.[29] Studies have also shown that treating mild thyroid conditions can increase the number of good-quality embryos in IVF.[30]

Thyroid antibodies are also very common in PCOS, with studies finding these antibodies in a quarter of women with PCOS.[31] Women with PCOS are also more likely to have hormonal imbalances indicative of underactive thyroid.

If you have a history of miscarriage, PCOS, unexplained infertility, an ovulation disorder, or premature ovarian failure, thyroid testing is particularly important. According to Dr. Amy Myers, a physician who specializes in thyroid disease, the most useful tests and optimal lab values are as follows:[32]

- TSH: 1.0–2.0 mIU/mL

- Free T4: at least 1.1 ng/dL

- Free T3: at least 3.2 pg/mL

- Reverse T3: less than a 10:1 ratio of reverse t3 to TSH

- Thyroid peroxidase antibodies: less than 9 IU/mL or negative

- Thyroglobulin antibodies: less than 4 IU/mL or negative

If your doctor is reluctant to run any thyroid tests, in most US states you can order these tests yourself through Life Extension or other online services that provide a requisition form for you to take to Quest or Labcorp. In the UK, tests can be ordered through Medichecks.

If a problem is detected, make an appointment with an endocrinologist so you can receive effective treatment. If your doctor does not appreciate the importance of carefully managing hypothyroidism in the context of infertility and miscarriage (and some may not), get a second opinion. Some endocrinologists consider a TSH below 4.5 mIU/mL to be "normal" and treatment at that level to be unnecessary, but many fertility specialists believe that closer to 1 mIU/mL is ideal.

In addition to prescribing replacement thyroid hormone, many endocrinologists will also recommend selenium supplementation and a gluten- and dairy-free diet in order to reduce the autoimmunity that causes poor thyroid function. For further information on these and other strategies to address root causes, I recommend Dr. Izabella Wentz's book *Hashimoto's Protocol* or Dr. Amy Myers's book *The Thyroid Connection*.

If you do have thyroid antibodies, it is also important to have your DHEA-S and testosterone levels tested. That is because women with thyroid autoimmunity are more likely to have a low level of the hormone DHEA, which is produced by the adrenals and is then converted into testosterone in the ovaries. This hormone is critical for early follicle development. If DHEA is low, as it often is in those with thyroid autoimmunity, egg development will be compromised. The result is what is often labeled as diminished ovarian reserve or premature ovarian insufficiency. As a result, it is very useful to ask your doctor to test your DHEA-S and testosterone levels. Correcting the problem by supplementing with DHEA (as discussed in chapter 9) can make the world of difference for some women with thyroid autoimmunity.

## Surprising Factor 3: Celiac Disease

Another factor that can occasionally contribute to infertility or miscarriage is celiac disease. This is an immune disorder in which gluten triggers the immune system to wage war on the body. The most well-known symptoms of celiac disease mimic irritable bowel syndrome, but many people with this condition do not actually show gastrointestinal symptoms.[33] Celiac disease can also manifest as anemia, headaches, fatigue, joint pain, skin disorders such as psoriasis, and a variety of other symptoms that differ widely between people.

Because celiac disease affects everyone differently, the condition often goes undiagnosed for many years. In Italy, celiac disease is taken very seriously, and all children are routinely screened for the disease by age six. But in the rest of the world, people with celiac disease often endure symptoms for many years before finding out the cause. By some reports, the average person with celiac disease visits five or more doctors before they are finally diagnosed, and in the United States it takes an average of five to 11 years to get a diagnosis.[34] Meanwhile, under the surface the immune system is waging war on the body, causing inflammation and damage.

One of the hallmarks of celiac disease is that the immune system severely damages the lining of the intestines, which in turn prevents proper absorption of nutrients. This inability to absorb nutrients leads to vitamin and mineral deficiencies that contribute to infertility.[35]

The link between celiac disease and infertility was first suggested in 1982.[36] Decades later, researchers are still grappling with the question of whether this condition is actually more prevalent in women with fertility problems.[37] In 2011, a study performed by Columbia University and Mayo Clinic found that celiac disease was no more common in a broad group of women with various types of infertility, but there was a significantly higher rate of celiac disease in women with *unexplained infertility*.[38] In that latter group, almost 6 percent of women had antibodies indicative of celiac disease, a rate that is about three times higher than the general population. This general pattern has now been reported in several other studies.[39]

More recently, a study of one thousand women undergoing IVF found that less that 2 percent had celiac antibodies, which is comparable to the usual frequency of celiac disease.[40] This fits with the previous research finding no increase in celiac disease in the general pool of infertility patients. Even so, this particular study has led to an even greater reluctance on the part of doctors to test for celiac disease in women having difficulty conceiving.

This reluctance is to some extent understandable. When looking at the research as a whole, it appears that celiac disease is only more common in cases that are truly unexplained. Even then, there is only a 5–8 percent chance that celiac disease is a factor. Nevertheless, testing might still be warranted if you would like to pursue a "no-stone-unturned approach," or if you have a family history of celiac disease or autoimmunity. (Celiac disease has a strong genetic component and many people with the condition develop other autoimmune diseases.)

Another scenario that may possibly justify testing is unexplained recurrent miscarriage. It is beyond controversy that miscarriages are more common in women with untreated celiac disease. One group of researchers found the miscarriage rate in women with untreated celiac disease to be almost nine times higher than in treated celiac patients.[41] Fortunately, adopting a gluten-free diet reverses much of this risk.

## Explaining the link between celiac, unexplained infertility, and miscarriage

Celiac disease likely contributes to infertility and miscarriage by both increasing inflammation and interfering with absorption of folate and other vitamins.[42] A reduction in folate in turn causes high homocysteine levels, which compromises egg quality and likely increases the risk of miscarriage.[43]

Excluding gluten allows the lining of the intestines to heal and restores the body's ability to absorb the nutrients that are critical to fertility. Just as we would hope, it appears that strictly following a gluten-free diet can start the process of rebalancing folate and homocysteine.[44]

Some researchers have found, however, that up to half of celiac patients carefully treated with a gluten-free diet still showed vitamin deficiencies. Specifically, many people with celiac disease who have followed a gluten-free diet for many years still have lower levels of folate and vitamin B6 and high levels of homocysteine.[45] But it appears that the situation can be improved with vitamin supplements.

When a large group of people with celiac disease were given a daily dose of folic acid, vitamin B12, and vitamin B6 for six months, their homocysteine levels returned to normal, and they reported significant improvements in well-being compared to those given a placebo.[46] This is not to say that a gluten-free diet should be ignored in favor of supplements, because celiac disease causes many other problems in addition to vitamin deficiencies, but rather suggests that prenatal vitamin supplements are likely to be even more important for people with celiac disease.

A significant proportion of celiacs also have elevated levels of a specific type of antibody known to cause miscarriage (antiphospholipid antibodies), but anecdotal reports suggest that these antibodies decline dramatically after adopting a strict gluten-free diet.[47] This is exactly what happened to one 34-year-old woman with antiphospholipid syndrome who suffered two miscarriages. Once diagnosed with celiac disease, she began a gluten-free diet, and within 6 months the previously elevated antibodies were undetectable.[48]

There also appears to be a link between celiac disease and thyroid autoimmunity, providing a further way in which this condition can impact fertility. It is now thought that 30–40 percent of people with celiac disease will also have a thyroid disorder, and celiac disease brings a threefold higher chance of developing thyroid disease.[49] As a practical matter, this means that if you have been found to have either thyroid disease or celiac disease, there is more reason to check for the other condition if you are struggling with infertility or miscarriage. A gluten-free diet may also help reduce the immune activity that drives thyroid disease.

The bottom line on celiac screening is that for most women, it is probably a lower priority than other tests. That is because it is only likely to be a factor in a small minority of cases. That said, there might be more reason to test for the condition if you have unexplained infertility, unexplained miscarriage, antiphospholipid antibody syndrome, thyroid disease, or a family history of celiac or autoimmunity.

## Surprising Factor 4: Dental Care

One additional factor that may impact your chance of conceiving and carrying to term is the health of your gums. For several years, researchers have seen evidence that gum disease significantly increases the risk of preterm birth and low birth weight.[50] A study published in the *Journal of the American Dental Association* reported that women with an advanced form of gum disease, called periodontitis, are four to seven times more likely to deliver prematurely.[51] Periodontitis also increases the risk of miscarriage.[52]

Gum disease is caused by bacteria building up between the teeth and gums, causing soreness and sometimes bleeding. The most common form of gum disease, called gingivitis, affects nearly half of women of childbearing age. If left untreated, this can progress to periodontitis, in which the gums start to pull away from the teeth, creating spaces called periodontal pockets that become infected. The infection causes an immune response that can result in inflammation spreading into the circulatory system.

The relationship between gum disease and miscarriage or premature birth is thought to be due to either the systemic inflammation that results from the bacterial infection or the bacteria from the gums making their way into amniotic fluid and causing a local immune response, which in turn increases the risk of miscarriage or premature birth.[53]

Yet the impact of gum disease does not end with miscarriage and premature birth—it may also increase the time it takes to get pregnant in the first place. This unexpected link was first revealed in 2011 by Dr. Roger Hart and a team of researchers at the University of Western Australia. As part of a larger study aiming to find out whether treating periodontal disease could improve pregnancy outcomes, the researchers screened more than three thousand pregnant women for periodontal disease, along with collecting information about how long it took each woman to conceive.[54]

The researchers found that on average, the women with periodontal disease took two months longer to conceive. Nearly a quarter of Caucasian women and 40 percent of non-Caucasian women were found to have periodontal disease, and these women took on average seven months to conceive, compared to five months for women without gum disease. Gum disease was also much more common in the women who had taken more than a year to conceive. As Dr. Hart suggested, these significant results indicate that all women should get a dental checkup before trying to conceive.

While it does not take much to get gum disease, it is also easy to prevent and reverse with regular flossing, brushing, and professional dental cleanings. Even fairly advanced periodontal disease can usually be resolved after less than four treatments by a periodontist.[55]

## Action Steps
### Basic, Intermediate, and Advanced Plans

If you have had difficulty getting pregnant or have lost one or more pregnancies to miscarriage, it may be worth testing for vitamin D deficiency, thyroid disease, and celiac disease. You should also get a dental checkup for gum disease.

Of these factors, thyroid testing should be considered the highest priority, while celiac screening is a lower priority in most cases. An alternative to testing your current vitamin D level is to add a vitamin D supplement, since the vast majority of women have vitamin D levels below the optimal range of 40 ng/mL (100 nmol/L). Many will need to supplement with 4000–5000 IU per day to reach this level.

**Part 2**

# HOW TO CHOOSE THE RIGHT SUPPLEMENTS

CHAPTER 5

# Prenatal Multivitamins

*"The more original a discovery, the more
obvious it seems afterwards."*
— ARTHUR KOESTLER

## Recommended for:
## Basic, Intermediate, and Advanced Fertility Plans

TAKING A PRENATAL multivitamin every day is one of the most important things you can do to prepare for pregnancy. And it is never too early to start. Vitamins such as folate are not only critical to preventing birth defects but may also make it easier to get pregnant, by restoring ovulation and boosting egg quality. Some vitamins can also help reduce the risk of miscarriage. For all these reasons, it is important to start taking a good-quality prenatal vitamin early—ideally at least three months before trying to conceive.

## Folate

Folate is a B vitamin needed throughout the body for hundreds of different biological processes. Folic acid is the synthetic form of folate used in supplements. This important vitamin is traditionally known for its role in preventing serious birth defects such as spina bifida, but recent research has also uncovered new evidence that folate plays a significant role even earlier—during the development of the egg. Because eggs begin maturing three to four months before ovulation, this suggests that the earlier you can start taking folate, the better.

It is not at all surprising that folate impacts egg quality, because it is important for making new DNA and proteins, along with playing a critical role in detoxification. Each of these processes plays an enormous role in early egg and embryo development. Before delving into the research showing that folate boosts fertility, it is useful to understand the broader context of how this vitamin came to be such an important part of planning for pregnancy.

Folic acid supplementation has now been hailed as one of the greatest public health achievements of the late twentieth century.[1] Yet it was not always so, and early research into the role of folic acid in preventing birth defects was marred by controversy. This controversy furnishes interesting background information for the other supplements discussed in this book because it provides an example of why there is often a huge gap between research findings and medical practice.

Until the 1990s, doctors had very little understanding of what could be done to prevent neural tube defects, which often resulted in stillbirth, death shortly after birth, or lifelong paralysis.

The world changed in 1991, when researchers in England published the results of a large study showing that 70–80 percent of neural tube defects could be prevented by taking a folic acid supplement immediately before pregnancy.[2] The beneficial effects of folic acid were so clear that the study was actually halted early so that more women could benefit from the findings.

Yet this large study was not the first to reveal that folic acid supplements could prevent neural tube defects. An earlier study showing the same thing,[3] published in 1981, generated many years of hostile criticism.[4]

The criticism mainly centered on the design of the trial because folic acid was given to all women presenting with a history of a previous pregnancy affected by neural tube defects, and the control group consisted of women who were already pregnant at the time they came to the doctors running the study. This is a departure from the ideal study design, in which a group of women are randomly assigned to receive either folic acid or a placebo, and the doctor and patient are "blind" as to which pill is being taken until the data are analyzed. This is referred to as a "gold standard" clinical trial and is designed to minimize the effect of bias.

In the case of folic acid, it was another 10 years before the results of the 1991 randomized, double-blind, placebo-controlled trial were available to confirm the initial research findings. In the meantime, the authors of the first study claimed that their results were persistently ignored while the possibility of a bias was overemphasized.[5] The practical impact of this controversy is that between 1981, when there was very good evidence of the protective effects of folic acid, and 1991, when a double-blind, placebo-controlled study finally satisfied the skeptics, 10 years passed, during which many women who should have been taking folic acid supplements were not, likely resulting in countless tragic outcomes that could have been prevented.

This serves as a cautionary tale that we should not overlook the best available evidence while we wait for the perfect clinical study—a philosophy echoed throughout this book. This philosophy of acting on the "best evidence" does of course need to be limited by safety concerns. If the benefit of a supplement is clear but we do not yet have reliable evidence of safety, it is absolutely necessary to wait for further research. But if safety has been firmly established in good-quality studies and there is good, but not perfect, evidence of a very significant benefit, we have every reason to act rather than waiting for a perfect clinical study that may never happen.

This is particularly true in the fertility context, in which women may have only one or two chances to conceive with IVF before running out of financial (or emotional) resources, and there is often no time to wait. That is the background for the supplement recommendations in the rest of this book: weighing all the available evidence for each supplement rather than waiting for medical practice to catch up with research.

Returning to the specific example of folic acid, we now know that taking this supplement before pregnancy dramatically cuts the risk of spina bifida and other neural tube defects.[6] The US Centers for Disease Control (CDC), the UK

Department of Health, and many other public health authorities recommend that to prevent neural tube defects, all women thinking of having a baby should take a 400 microgram (0.4 milligram) folic acid supplement every day, in addition to natural dietary sources of folate.[7]

This should be considered a minimum, and some authorities recommend at least 800 micrograms for all women trying to conceive. As will be discussed further below, it is also preferable to choose a prenatal that contains a natural form of folate, such as methylfolate, rather than synthetic folic acid.

Preventing birth defects is not the only reason to begin taking a prenatal multivitamin before pregnancy. Another benefit of starting early is that vitamins such as folate may help you conceive sooner and prevent miscarriage. The latest research clearly establishes that folate is important for every stage of fertility, from egg development to ovulation to fetal growth.[8]

## Folate and Ovulation

Doctors have long suspected that vitamin deficiencies could play a role in ovulation problems in some women. This idea was supported by the results of the Nurses Health Study, which followed thousands of nurses over many years. The second round of the study followed a subgroup of more than 18,000 women trying to conceive or who became pregnant, with no history of infertility, over eight years.

When researchers at the Harvard School of Public Health analyzed the data from the Nurses Health Study, they found that the women who took a daily multivitamin were much less likely to have infertility due to ovulation problems. Taking a multivitamin just a few times per week was associated with a one-third lower chance of ovulatory infertility, and women who took a multivitamin every day had an even lower risk.[9] The researchers suggested that this was probably due to folic acid and other B vitamins.

The link between multivitamin use and fertility had actually been seen before in smaller studies in which researchers concluded that taking a multivitamin improves fertility.[10] These double-blind studies found higher pregnancy rates in women taking a multivitamin than women taking a placebo.

A diet higher in folate also increases progesterone levels and reduces the risk of ovulation disorders.[11] In one study, the third of women with the highest consumption of folate from fortified grains had a 65 percent lower chance of ovulation disorders and had higher levels of progesterone at the time needed for optimal fertility.[12]

## Folate and Egg Quality

Folate also appears to improve egg quality and IVF success rates. Women who take folic acid supplements before IVF have also been found to have higher-quality eggs, and a higher proportion of mature eggs, than women not taking additional folate.[13] As a result, researchers have reported that women with a twofold higher level of folate in ovarian follicles were three times more likely to become pregnant.[14]

### Synthetic folic acid versus methylfolate

If you have a history of infertility or recurrent miscarriage, one possible culprit is a genetic variation that reduces your ability to metabolize folate. A 2016 study by researchers at Oxford University found that women with certain variants in the folate metabolism gene, MTHFR, were more likely to have chromosomally abnormal embryos and implantation failure and were much less likely to become pregnant following IVF.[15] These variants have also long been associated with recurrent miscarriage,[16] although some recent studies have questioned this link.[17]

The enzyme encoded by the MTHFR gene is responsible for converting other forms of folate to the biologically active form, methylfolate. Methylfolate has many key roles, but perhaps its most important is detoxification. The body uses methylfolate to detoxify unwanted byproducts of normal metabolism, such as homocysteine.

Certain common variations in the MTHFR gene reduce the activity of the enzyme that produces methylfolate from other forms of folate. This reduces the amount of methylfolate available for detoxification functions, which allows homocysteine to accumulate. It is in fact the excess of homocysteine that is thought to contribute to infertility and possibly miscarriage risk in those with MTHFR mutations.[18] High homocysteine not only contributes to DNA damage but may also increase the risk of blood clots (although this issue is controversial).

The two most common variants in the MTHFR gene are known as A1298C and C677T. Approximately 40 percent of the population has one copy of A1298C, but this causes only a mild reduction in the ability to process folate (a 20–40 percent reduction in enzyme activity). Having two copies of this variant, or having one or two copies of the C677T variant, has a much more significant impact, reducing the activity of the enzyme by up to 70 percent. These more signficant muta-tions affect approximately 10 percent of the population and are associated with higher homocysteine levels.[19]

There is currently a heated debate on the extent to which these mutations contribute to recurrent miscarriage. Some studies have found a connection, while others have not.[20] The good news is that if MTHFR variants do indeed increase the risk of miscarriage, it appears that much of this risk can be mitigated with the right supplements.

If you would like to know your genotype, your doctor can order a MTHFR blood test, or you can order DNA analysis yourself through 23andme then upload your data to the free website GeneticGenie.org. Testing is not essential, though, because you can simply choose to supplement as you would if the mutations were present.

Historically, doctors have recommended that women with an MTHFR mutation should take a much higher dose of folic acid (1000–4000 mcg) to make up for the reduced efficiency of processing folic acid to methylfolate. It is now known that this leads to an accumulation of unmetabolized folic acid in the bloodstream, which appears to interfere with the ability of cells to take up methylfolate.[21] A much more effective approach is to supplement directly with methylfolate.[22] (Recommended prenatals that contain folate in this form are listed at www. itstartswiththeegg.com.)

If you have not yet had any genetic testing, but you have a history of recurrent miscarriage or failed IVF cycles, the most cautious approach is to take a prenatal with folate in the form of methylfolate, just in case you do have a mutation that compromises folate metabolism. It may also make sense for your partner to take a methylfolate supplement, because new research indicates that when a father has defects in folate metabolism, this may also contribute to miscarriage, likely by increasing DNA damage within sperm.[23]

The typical recommended dose of methylfolate for those with MTHFR variants is 800–1000 micrograms per day. In rare cases, methylfolate does, however, cause side effects in some people. Possible side effects include muscle pain, anxiety, or other mood changes.

If you find that methylfolate bothers you, one option is getting tested for MTHFR variants to see if you really need this form of folate. If you have no variant or only one copy of the A1298C variant (which about 40 percent of the population have), you have more options with the choice of prenatal vitamins. Dr. Ben Lynch, author of *Dirty Genes* and an expert on MTHFR mutations, also recommends supplementing with vitamin B12 in the form of hydroxocobalamin for those who experience side effects from methylfolate.

Taking more vitamin B12 has the added advantage of further reducing homocysteine levels. As a result, initial studies have suggested that this vitamin may be just as important as folate in preventing miscarriages associated with MTHFR variants.[24]

## Prenatals for those without MTHFR mutations

If testing shows that you do not have a significant mutation in the MTHFR gene, it may still be preferable to choose a prenatal that contains methylfolate or another natural form of folate, rather than synthetic folic acid. That is because the processing of synthetic folic acid is not very efficient and varies significantly between people, even without MTHFR variants.

It used to be thought that humans quickly converted synthetic folic acid into other forms, because that is what happens in rodents. Yet recent studies show that in humans, a substantial amount of synthetic folic acid remains unmetabolized and unable to be used.[25] If it accumulates in high levels, it may interfere with the uptake of methylfolate,[26] which cells need for a variety of important functions.

There are other versions of folate naturally found in foods, such as folinic acid, that are quickly converted to usable methylfolate.[27] Given the critical importance of folate to ovulation, egg quality, and preventing miscarriage, the last thing anyone needs is a low folate level due to poor conversion of synthetic folic acid.

It is therefore preferable to choose a prenatal that contains either natural food folate (which is typically obtained from lemon peels), folinic acid, or methylfolate, even if you do not have significant MTHFR variants. The total amount of folate should be at least 800 micrograms. If your prenatal contains less, it is a good idea to supplement with an additional 400 micrograms of folinic acid (also known as calcium folinate) or methylfolate.

See **www.itstartswiththeegg.com** for current prenatal recommendations.

## Other Vitamins and Fertility

A typical prenatal multivitamin will contain several other vitamins that are also important for fertility. One that plays a particularly critical role in egg quality is vitamin B12. In the same

Dutch study investigating the role of folate in women undergoing IVF, researchers found that high levels of vitamin $B_{12}$ are also associated with better embryo quality. This is likely because vitamin $B_{12}$, like folate, decreases homocysteine.[28]

Another specific vitamin that may improve fertility is vitamin B6. In 2007, Dr. Alayne Ronnenberg and scientists from the University of Illinois, Harvard Medical School, and Northwestern University published a study showing that women with low levels of vitamin B6 were less likely to become pregnant and more likely to miscarry.

All of this research indicates that taking a prenatal multivitamin that includes sufficient methylfolate, vitamin B12, and vitamin B6 could make it much easier for you to become pregnant and reduce the risk of miscarriage and birth defects.

The minerals found in prenatal multivitamins may also be important during the time before pregnancy. For example, zinc, selenium, and iodine are necessary for proper thyroid function. This has implications for fertility because an underactive thyroid gland may suppress ovulation and raise the risk of miscarriage. Zinc and selenium are also involved in antioxidant defense systems and so likely play a role in egg quality, as discussed in the next chapter.

## An Introduction to Other Supplements

The next several chapters will describe other specific supplements that you can take in addition to your prenatal multivitamin to improve egg quality. If you are going to add just one other supplement, make it Coenzyme Q10 (CoQ10 for short). As explained in the next chapter, the latest research suggests that taking CoQ10 increases egg and embryo quality by increasing the supply of cellular energy available to eggs.

The subsequent chapters discuss additional supplements that may improve egg quality in women who are trying to conceive after 35, as well as women who have a history of infertility or previous miscarriages.

By way of general overview, chapter 6 on CoQ10 and chapter 7 on antioxidants are generally applicable to anyone trying to conceive. Chapter 8 on myo-inositol is more relevant to women with PCOS, irregular ovulation, or a history of miscarriage and insulin resistance. Chapter 9 on DHEA is relevant for women with diminished ovarian reserve, autoimmunity, age-related infertility, or a history of miscarriage. Chapter 10 discusses why some so-called "fertility supplements" are best avoided, while chapter 11 covers supplements that may be useful while preparing for frozen embryo transfer.

**CHAPTER 6**

# Energize Your Eggs with Coenzyme Q10

*"Energy and persistence conquer all things."*
— BENJAMIN FRANKLIN

### Recommended for
### Basic, Intermediate, and Advanced Fertility Plans

COENZYME Q10, OR CoQ10 for short, is a small molecule found in just about every cell in the body, including your eggs. Recent scientific research has revealed just how important this molecule is to preserving egg quality and fertility. Along with many other benefits, adding a CoQ10 supplement may have the potential to prevent or even reverse some of the decline in egg quality that comes with age.

Anyone trying to conceive can likely benefit from adding a CoQ10 supplement, but it is particularly helpful if you are in your mid-30s or older, or have fertility problems such as diminished ovarian reserve.

## What Does CoQ10 Do?

CoQ10 has long been a favorite nutritional supplement of marathon runners and Olympic athletes,[1] and a standard recommended supplement to prevent the muscle pain associated with cholesterol-lowering statin drugs. CoQ10 has also shown some initial promise in large clinical studies on a range of conditions that include congestive heart failure, Parkinson's, Huntington's, and Lou Gehrig's disease. But research has recently suggested yet another likely benefit of CoQ10: improved egg quality.

How is it that one tiny molecule can do so much? It is probably because CoQ10 plays such an important role in making energy throughout the body—in muscles, the brain, and developing eggs. CoQ10 is in fact critical for energy production by the power plants inside our cells, mitochondria.

CoQ10 plays a direct role inside mitochondria by transferring electrons between other molecules. In other words, CoQ10 is a vital part of the "electron transport chain" that creates electrical energy (i.e., voltage) inside mitochondria. The mitochondria harness this electrical energy to make energy in the form of ATP. Cells then use ATP as the fuel to power just about every biological process.

CoQ10 is also an antioxidant that can recycle vitamin E and perform many other roles inside cells,[2] but it is the role this molecule plays in mitochondria that is most interesting for improving egg quality.

To understand how taking a CoQ10 supplement can

improve egg quality, we first need to examine how poor egg quality relates to the supply of cellular energy and why this energy supply is compromised in the eggs of older women.

## Energy for Eggs

As we age, mitochondria become damaged and are less efficient energy producers, much like an old, damaged power plant.[3] This decline in mitochondrial function is actually thought to play a key role in the aging process[4] and happens throughout the body, but particularly in eggs. Studies have specifically shown that in eggs from women over 40, structural damage to mitochondria is much more common.[5] Aging eggs also accumulate genetic damage in mitochondria,[6] and even the number of mitochondria decline in the follicle cells that surround each egg.[7]

As a result, mitochondria in eggs from older women make less energy—that is, less ATP.[8] The inability to make enough ATP is a big problem for egg quality and is likely a major way in which age negatively effects egg quality.[9]

But poorly functioning mitochondria are not just relevant to age-related infertility. There is also evidence of poor mitochondrial function in women with other fertility concerns, such as premature ovarian failure or a poor response to stimulation medication in IVF.[10]

A pioneer in this research, Dr. Jonathan Van Blerkom, first suggested in 1995 that there is a link between the ATP level in an egg and that egg's potential to mature properly and become a high-quality embryo.[11] This has since been confirmed by several researchers who have demonstrated that an egg's ability to produce a spike of ATP in the specific time and place needed for major developmental tasks is absolutely critical for proper egg development.[12]

It is now a generally accepted principle that having high-performing mitochondria is a hallmark of egg quality.[13] According to leading researchers in the field, the ability to make energy when needed is the single most important factor in determining the competence of eggs and embryos.[14] The better an egg's ability to produce energy, the more likely it is to mature and successfully fertilize.[15]

There is also a growing body of direct evidence that the ability of an egg to produce energy when needed is particularly important to being able to mature with the correct number of chromosomes. This is because the process of separating and ejecting chromosomes is very energy-intensive.[16] Scientists have actually seen the mitochondria cluster together and suddenly produce a burst of ATP at the precise time and place needed to form the structure that separates the chromosomes.[17]

If an egg does not have enough energy to neatly organize the chromosomes and separate the set of chromosomes to be pushed out, it may end up with an incorrect number of chromosome copies and will become an embryo with little chance of survival.

Just as we would expect, research has found that human embryos with poorly functioning mitochondria are more likely to have disrupted chromosomal processing machinery and chaotic chromosome distribution.[18] In addition, other researchers have shown that if mitochondria in mouse eggs are intentionally damaged, the ATP level goes down, and the machinery that separates chromosomes disassembles and malfunctions.[19]

As discussed in earlier chapters, errors in the number of

chromosome copies are the single greatest cause of failure of embryos to survive the first week, implantation failure, and early pregnancy loss. Chromosomal errors become much more common after the midthirties and are also more common in people with a history of fertility problems or several early miscarriages. Suboptimal energy production by mitochondria may therefore directly contribute to infertility, failed IVF cycles, and early pregnancy loss by contributing to chromosome segregation errors in eggs.[20]

But energy supply is not just important for proper chromosomal processing—it also provides the fuel for the growing embryo. Problems with energy production in an egg can manifest later in embryo development because ATP is needed for all the work an embryo must do to grow to the blastocyst stage and successfully implant.[21] Dysfunctional mitochondria in eggs are thought to be especially problematic for early embryo survival.[22]

## CoQ10 to Improve Egg Quality

Based on all the scientific knowledge about the importance of fully functioning mitochondria to egg and embryo quality, it stands to reason that anything we can do to boost mitochondrial function and help eggs produce more energy will improve egg quality and embryo viability. Research suggests that CoQ10 does just that.

As explained by Dr. Yaakov Bentov, a fertility specialist who has pioneered the use of CoQ10 to improve egg quality, "our thought is that it's not the egg that's different [in older women]; it's the ability of the egg to produce the kind of energy needed to complete all the processes that are involved with maturing and being fertilized. That's why we're recommending that women use all these supplements like co-enzyme Q10."[23]

CoQ10 has powerful benefits because it is an essential raw ingredient needed for energy production by mitochondria.[24] Many studies have shown that adding CoQ10 to cells grown in the laboratory increases the production of ATP.[25] It has also been found to protect mitochondria from damage.[26]

CoQ10 is naturally found in ovarian follicles to perform this important role of supporting energy production and protecting mitochondria. Researchers have even measured the amount of CoQ10 naturally present inside follicles. What they found will probably come as no surprise: a higher level of CoQ10 is associated with higher-quality eggs and a higher pregnancy rate.[27]

In the fertility context, the thinking is that by taking a CoQ10 supplement to increase the supply of this important nutrient, we can increase the energy supply needed to fuel egg development. This would be expected to prevent chromosomal errors and increase egg and embryo viability.

When this book was first published in 2014, the idea of improving egg quality with CoQ10 was relatively new. There was a clear scientific rationale for using the supplement, based on the pioneering research of Dr. Bentov and his colleague, Dr. Robert Casper (the founder of TRIO fertility in Toronto).[28] Yet there was still a lack of controlled studies confirming that it would work.

In 2018, two controlled studies were published confirming that taking CoQ10 for one or two months before IVF does significantly boost egg quality.[29] In those women taking CoQ10, more eggs fertilized and there was a higher proportion of good-quality embryos. Perhaps the most significant difference was in the number of cancelled cycles and the number of embryos available to freeze. In the women taking CoQ10, only 8 percent of cycles were cancelled due to poor egg development, compared to 23 percent of controls. Additionally, 18 percent of women from the CoQ10 group had embryos available to freeze, compared to 4 percent of those in the control group.

A double-blind, placebo-controlled study by Dr. Bentov and Dr. Casper also found a lower rate of chromosomal abnormalities in embryos from women taking CoQ10.[30]

## Supplementing with CoQ10

CoQ10 is made in just about every cell in the body, but as we age, the body may not be able to make enough CoQ10 to keep up with the demands to make cellular energy. It is extremely difficult to obtain significant amounts from food, so adding a supplement is the best solution.

In the clinical trials conducted so far, the dose ranged from 400–600 milligrams per day of CoQ10, starting one or two months before IVF. This is actually a fairly conservative dose, with studies outside the fertility context reporting safety of much higher doses. A recent double-blind study reported no safety concerns with 2400 milligrams taken daily for five years.[31]

To benefit egg quality, the minimum dose likely depends on the precise form of CoQ10 used. The standard form in supplements is called ubiquinone. This form is not very soluble, so much of it is not absorbed. What does get absorbed is then converted (in chemistry-speak, "reduced") to the second form of CoQ10 to become an active antioxidant. This second form is called ubiquinol. More than 95 percent of the CoQ10 in circulation is in this reduced ubiquinol form.[32]

To get around the problem of poorly absorbed ubiquinone, it is possible to buy a supplement already in the form of ubiquinol. Good-quality brands include Jarrow Ubiquinol QH Absorb.

Even though ubiquinol is typically more expensive than traditional CoQ10, it may still offer better value because you can take a lower dose and will absorb significantly more of the active ingredient.[33]

Another option is to choose a special formulation of ubiquinone that is designed to be more readily absorbed. A variety of solutions have been developed to formulate ubiquinone in a way that increases absorption, such as suspending it in tiny droplets.[34]

Studies have shown that some of these high-tech formulations are absorbed significantly better than traditional ubiquinone supplements.[35] Recommended brands include Bio-Quinon and Qunol Ultra CoQ10.

Bio-Quinon, which is manufactured in Denmark by Pharma Nord, may even be more readily absorbed than ubiquinol. That was the finding of a study published in the journal *Nutrition* in 2019. Researchers tested seven different supplement formulations containing 100 mg of CoQ10 in 14 young, healthy individuals.[36] They found that the two formulations that were best at raising CoQ10 levels in the body were ubiquinol Kaneka QH (found in Jarrow's Ubiquinol, for instance) and a particular soft-gel version of ubiquinone in a soy oil matrix, made by Pharma Nord.

This second version is sold under the name Myoqinon in Europe and Bio-Quinon Q10 Gold in the United States. Participants absorbed more than twice as much CoQ10 from these formulations compared to the other supplements.

This study, which was supported by Pharma Nord, suggested

that their own brand of CoQ10 was actually absorbed even better than ubiquinol, although there was evidence suggesting that ubiquinol was retained in cells longer.

Pharma-Nord's CoQ10 was actually the specific form used in one of the 2018 studies showing an improvement in egg quality, and it has now become widely recommended by fertility clinics. Yet using this form is by no means essential. The other studies using conventional CoQ10 also show a benefit, albeit at a higher dose, and we know that ubiquinol is also readily absorbed and highly effective. For a comparison of the dose and brands used in clinical trials in the IVF context, see the table following:

| Study | Form | Brand | Total Daily Dose |
|---|---|---|---|
| Casper (2014) | Ubiquinone, micronized | Advanced Orthomolecular Research | 600 mg, once per day |
| Gianubillo (2018) | Ubiquinone, improved absorption | Pharma Nord Bio-Quinon | 400mg (divided into 2 doses) |
| Xu (2018) | Ubiquinone, standard | GNC | 600 mg (divided into 3 doses) |

Based on these studies, the recommended dose for those trying to conceive through IVF, or with a history of miscarriage or infertility, is 400 mg of Bio-Quinon or 400 mg of ubiquinol. Alternatively, you may decide to take 600 mg of standard CoQ10, although studies outside the IVF context indicate that this will be less effective than the recommended formulations. Some IVF clinics now take an even more aggressive approach and recommend 600 mg of Bio-Quinon or ubiquinol. There is likely little downside to this higher dose, other than additional cost.

If you are just beginning the process of trying to conceive and have no reason to expect fertility problems, a lower dose of 200 mg of ubiquinol or Bio-Quinon is probably sufficient.

In addition to choosing one of the preferred forms of CoQ10, you can also maximize the benefit by dividing the dose. That is because there is a limit to how much can be absorbed at a time, with the percentage absorbed beginning to drop when the dose is above 200 mg. If you are taking 400 mg per day, it is therefore helpful to take the supplement in two separate doses—one 200 mg capsule with breakfast and another capsule with lunch.[37] (Some people experience trouble sleeping when CoQ10 is taken at night.) CoQ10 is fat soluble and therefore best absorbed with meals.

## Safety and Side Effects

Because CoQ10 holds promise in treating a range of diseases associated with impaired mitochondrial function, it has been studied extensively in large clinical trials. As part of these double-blind, placebo-controlled clinical studies, thousands of people have taken ubiquinone CoQ10 at high doses over many years and have been carefully observed. Researchers have reported no safety concerns, even at doses as high as 3000 mg/day.[38] At the time of writing, the only significant side effect reported in clinical studies is mild gastrointestinal symptoms in a small number of people.[39]

Because studies have found that CoQ10 helps to lower high blood pressure, those with blood pressure that is lower than normal may be reluctant to take this supplement. You should talk to your doctor about this, but bear in mind that the ability to bring high blood pressure down does not necessarily mean CoQ10 will also reduce already normal or low pressure.

A 2018 study of orthostatic hypotension (when blood pressure drops with standing) found that the supplement actually improved the condition and helped prevent reductions in blood pressure.[40] This suggests that at least in some cases of low blood pressure, CoQ10 is not problematic and may in fact help. (Low blood pressure is likely more common in those with fertility issues, because both can stem from adrenal dysfunction, discussed further in the chapter on DHEA.)

One possible effect of CoQ10 to be aware of is that it has been reported to gradually improve blood sugar control in people with type 2 diabetes,[41] although studies on this point have been inconsistent.[42] If you have diabetes, it is a good idea to discuss your plan to start taking CoQ10 with your doctor. Eventually your doctor may be able to reduce the dose of your diabetes medication.

## When to Start and When to Stop

Whether you are trying to conceive naturally, or with the help of IUI or IVF, it is best to start taking CoQ10 as early as possible. Ideally, at least three months before a planned IUI or IVF cycle. Because it takes approximately three months for eggs to fully develop, supplementing throughout this window of time allows the eggs to mature in an optimal environment, with a good supply of energy to process chromosomes correctly. Nevertheless, the most recent clinical studies show that even taking CoQ10 for one or two months before IVF can be very helpful.

Different doctors provide different advice on when to stop taking CoQ10. If you are trying to conceive naturally or through IUI, it is typical to stop taking CoQ10 when you get a positive pregnancy test. In the context of IVF, many clinics recommend stopping CoQ10 and other egg-quality supplements the day before egg retrieval, since the supplements are no longer needed. Others advise stopping when you get a positive pregnancy test, so that you can continue to benefit from the supplement if you end up needing to do another cycle. Continuing to take CoQ10 after egg retrieval could also potentially help prepare the uterine lining for embryo transfer, as discussed in chapter 11.

Ultimately, the precise timing probably does not matter all that much, but a reasonable middle-ground approach is to stop taking the supplement after embryo transfer while you wait to find out if the transfer is successful. If you do not get pregnant, then you can restart the supplement and will have only had a two-week break.

Keep in mind that doctors advise patients to stop taking CoQ10 during pregnancy simply because 0f a lack of data. There have not been any large studies demonstrating safety during pregnancy, and doctors are understandably extremely conservative about supplements during this time. Yet there is little reason to expect that taking CoQ10 while pregnant is harmful. To the contrary, research so far indicates that CoQ10 may actually be able to reduce the risk of preeclampsia. (This is a serious complication of pregnancy that involves danger-ously high blood pressure.)

One specific circumstance in which there may be a justifica-tion for taking a small amount of CoQ10 during early pregnancy (acknowledging that there is a lack of safety data) is recurrent miscarriage. When researchers measured the CoQ10 levels in almost five hundred pregnant women, they found that levels normally rise with each trimester. Yet another trend was evident too: Those women with low levels were more likely to miscarry.

The reason for this is unclear, but new research suggests at least one interesting link between CoQ10 and miscarriage that goes beyond egg quality. Specifically, CoQ10 appears to reduce the immune and clotting mediators involved in antiphospho-lipid syndrome, a common cause of miscarriage. In a random-ized, placebo-controlled study published in 2017, 36 patients with antiphospholipid syndrome were randomized to receive 200 mg/day of ubiquinol, or a placebo.[13] After one month there was a significant reduction in the immune and clot-ting mediators involved in antiphospholipid syndrome. We do not know how this would translate to miscarriage, but it is a promising avenue of research.

## Conclusion

Given everything we know about how CoQ10 increases energy production in mitochondria, how important this energy pro-duction is for egg and embryo development, and the positive results from clinical studies to date, the current evidence sug-gests that adding a CoQ10 supplement is one of the best ways to improve egg quality.

# CHAPTER 7

# Melatonin and Other Antioxidants

*"All truth passes through three stages: First, it is ridiculed; second, it is violently opposed; third, it is accepted as self-evident."*
—ARTHUR SCHOPENHAUER

## Recommended for:
## Intermediate and Advanced Fertility Plans

ANTIOXIDANTS PLAY A vital role in egg quality by protecting against a condition known as oxidative stress. Although ovarian follicles naturally contain a whole host of antioxidant vitamins and enzymes, these are often diminished in women with unexplained infertility, PCOS, and age-related infertility.

If you are young and healthy, with no fertility issues, a prenatal multivitamin and healthy diet (more on that in chapter 13) will likely provide all the antioxidants you need. But if you are in your midthirties or older, have specific fertility challenges, or a history of miscarriage, you may need an additional antioxidant supplement to optimize egg quality.

## What Are Antioxidants?

Antioxidants have long been known to play a role in fertility. The chemical name for vitamin E, tocopherol, was actually based on this important role, coming from the Greek word "tocos," meaning "childbirth," and "phero," meaning "to bring forth."[1] But vitamin E is just one of many antioxidants involved in fertility.

Some explanation of the terminology is useful to set the stage. The term "antioxidant" refers to a molecule that neutralizes reactive oxygen molecules. Reactive oxygen molecules are formed during normal metabolism and include "free radicals," which are particularly reactive because each oxygen molecule has an unpaired electron. The problem with reactive oxygen molecules, such as free radicals, is that when they react with other molecules, they cause oxidation.

The process of oxidation can be seen in everyday life, such as when metal rusts or silver tarnishes. Analogous chemical reactions occur inside cells. If not kept in check, oxidation can damage DNA, proteins, lipids, cell membranes, and mitochondria. But that is where antioxidants come in—they can be considered protectors against this chemical reaction of oxidation, analogous to using lemon juice to prevent an apple from turning brown.

Because of the potential of oxidants to cause cellular damage, each cell has an army of antioxidant defenses, including antioxidant enzymes produced with the specific purpose of neutralizing free radicals. Other important components of the antioxidant defense system are vitamins A, C, and E. Each of these antioxidants is found in developing eggs and has a role to play in preventing oxidative damage.

## How Do Antioxidants Impact Egg Quality?

As we age, oxidative damage causes more and more problems for eggs.[2] This is in part due to a weakened antioxidant enzyme defense system in aging eggs; in eggs from older women, researchers have seen reduced production of antioxidant enzymes, which leaves more oxidizing molecules free to cause damage.[3] Unfortunately, eggs from older women also produce more oxidizing molecules to begin with because aging mitochondria "leak" electrons when they become damaged, which creates reactive oxidizing molecules.[4]

Mitochondria, those tiny power plants in every cell in the body, are actually a major source of reactive oxygen molecules and also a major victim.[5] Mitochondria are particularly sensitive to oxidative damage and release more oxidants when damaged, causing a vicious cycle resulting in more damage and more free radicals.[6]

All this oxidative damage to mitochondria reduces their ability to produce cellular energy in the form of ATP—energy that is critically important to egg development and embryo viability. Oxidative damage to mitochondria is now thought to be one of the major ways that aging impacts egg quality.

This oxidative damage is not limited to eggs from older women. Researchers have also found reduced antioxidant enzyme levels and higher levels of reactive oxygen molecules in women with unexplained infertility.[7] In one recent study, 70 percent of women with unexplained premature ovarian failure had elevated oxidation levels.[8] Even in eggs from young mice, oxidative stress decreases energy production and destabilizes chromosome processing.[9]

As a brief side note, an increased level of oxidative stress has also been seen in women with a history of PCOS, miscarriage, preeclampsia, and endometriosis.[10]

In the specific case of endometriosis, the precise role of oxidative stress and poor egg quality in contributing to infertility remains controversial.[11] Several studies have found that in women undergoing IVF, endometriosis only reduces the number of eggs retrieved (possible reasons for this will be discussed in the chapter on DHEA), without any major impact on egg quality. Some have reported that the eggs obtained from women with endometriosis are just as likely to lead to a healthy pregnancy as for any other IVF patient.[12] But other studies have indicated a reduction in egg quality associated with endometriosis.[13]

If egg quality truly is a component of infertility in endometriosis, new research indicates that this may be due to oxidative damage. Two studies published in 2018 reported higher levels of oxidative damage in the follicles of women with endometriosis.[14] One of these studies also found that when oxidation levels were higher, there was a lower chance of an egg making it to the blastocyst stage.

In women with PCOS, the role of oxidative stress is even clearer. The condition often involves insulin resistance and high blood sugar. As a result of this high blood sugar, the body produces more reactive oxygen molecules, which increases oxidative stress.[15] (For the same reason, controlling blood sugar levels through diet, as discussed in chapter 13, is particularly helpful in limiting oxidative stress at the source.)

Adding to this problem of increased oxidants in PCOS is the fact that PCOS is also associated with a decline in antioxidant activity.[16] As a result of these two hits, women with PCOS have higher levels of oxidation, which is thought to damage mitochondria and disrupt chromosome processing.[17] Poor egg quality as a result of oxidative stress is likely a major component of fertility problems in PCOS.[18]

The scientific research is also clear that eggs and embryos from older women, and women with fertility problems, have reduced antioxidant defense systems and are more sensitive to oxidative damage.[19] This oxidative damage is believed to damage mitochondria, compromising energy production and egg quality.[20]

Fortunately, antioxidants may be able to prevent some of this damage,[21] with the net effect of improving fertility.[22] Researchers have found that women with higher total antioxidant levels during IVF cycles have a greater chance of becoming pregnant.[23] Most recently, a large study of women undergoing fertility treatment at Boston IVF and Harvard Vanguard Medical Associates concluded that the use of antioxidant supplements was associated with a shorter time to pregnancy.[24] While there is still much more to investigate and many conflicting results so far, the balance of the current evidence suggests that having well-armed antioxidant defenses can protect eggs and improve fertility.

When it comes to determining which specific antioxidant supplements are most useful for fertility, initial research suggests that the best options are vitamin C, vitamin E, alpha-lipoic acid, N-acetylcysteine, and melatonin. Each of these supplements serves slightly different purposes and may suit different situations, as the remainder of this chapter explains.

## Melatonin

Melatonin is a hormone secreted at night by a small gland deep inside the brain, the pineal gland. You may know it as a natural sleep aid. Melatonin is used for this purpose because it regulates circadian rhythms, telling the body to go to sleep at night and wake up in the morning. It is so important in regulating sleep that exposure to bright light at night, which suppresses melatonin production in the brain, can compromise sleep quality and cause insomnia.

Melatonin is not just a sleep regulator, though—it is also involved in fertility. In some species, melatonin is involved in regulating seasonal fertility to ensure that lambs, calves, and other baby animals are born in spring.[25] Melatonin also plays a surprisingly important role in human fertility.

One clue that melatonin is important to human fertility is that particularly high levels of melatonin are found in the fluid of ovarian follicles.[26] Also, the amount of melatonin in the follicle fluid increases as the follicles grow. This was observed in women undergoing IVF, where higher levels of melatonin were found in larger, developed follicles than in small follicles.[27]

Researchers have suggested that the increased level of melatonin as follicles grow has an important role in ovulation.[28]

## Melatonin and fertility

What exactly melatonin does in the ovaries is still not fully understood. Melatonin has traditionally been regarded as a hormonal messenger molecule that works by binding to specific receptors and thereby sending a message to cells. In other words, it was thought of as a molecule that merely communicates rather than having a direct biological effect. But in 1993, it was discovered that melatonin is also a powerful antioxidant that directly neutralizes free radicals.[29] This has since been confirmed by many different studies.[30] In some ways, melatonin is an even more powerful antioxidant than vitamin C and vitamin E.[31]

Unfortunately, melatonin levels decline with age,[32] and as a result, the ovaries lose this natural protector against oxidative stress. In 2017 and 2018, two separate groups of researchers discovered a significant correlation between melatonin levels in ovarian follicles and markers of ovarian reserve.[33]

Women with higher melatonin levels had higher anti-mullerian hormone (AMH) and a higher follicle count. There was also a correlation between melatonin levels and the results of IVF cycles, with higher melatonin levels corresponding to a greater number of eggs retrieved, and more high-quality embryos after IVF. The study also found that melatonin levels declined with age.

A reduction in melatonin could therefore be one contributor to age-related infertility, but it is also a factor that can be changed. There is clear evidence that melatonin supplement can restore antioxidant defenses inside eggs and improve egg quality.

Over the past 20 years, an array of animal and laboratory studies have demonstrated that melatonin helps eggs to mature properly and develop into good-quality embryos, in part due to antioxidant activity.[34] All these studies led doctors to believe that melatonin may also improve egg and embryo quality in women undergoing IVF. And so the human clinical trials began.

In one of the first studies giving melatonin to women undergoing IVF, researchers found that melatonin lowered levels of oxidative stress and cellular oxidative damage in ovarian follicles—a very promising discovery.[35] Researchers then found that supplementing with melatonin not only reduces oxidative damage but also improves egg and embryo quality.

In a study led by Dr. Hiroshi Tamura, nine women were given melatonin from the beginning of an IVF cycle, and their egg quality was compared to each woman's previous cycle. After treatment with melatonin, there was a dramatic improvement, with an average of 65 percent of their eggs giving rise to good-quality embryos, compared to just 27 percent in the previous cycle.[36]

The next step was to investigate the impact of melatonin on the actual pregnancy rate in IVF to see if melatonin really increased the chance of becoming pregnant. To that end, Dr. Tamura and a group of doctors in Japan performed a trailblazing clinical study involving 115 women who had a previous failed IVF cycle and a low fertilization rate.[37] Before undertaking another IVF cycle, half the women were given melatonin. These women went on to have a fertilization rate much higher than the previous cycle, and nearly 20 percent of the melatonin-treated women became pregnant.

By contrast, the women not given melatonin had the same low fertilization rate as their previous cycle, and only 10 percent of these women became pregnant. These results demonstrated that melatonin improved the fertilization rate and nearly doubled the chance of becoming pregnant through IVF.

Dr. Tamura noted: "Our study represents the first clinical application of melatonin treatment for infertility patients. This work needs to be confirmed, but we believe that melatonin treatment is likely to become a significant option for improving oocyte quality in women who cannot become pregnant because of poor oocyte quality."[38]

The ability of melatonin supplements to improve egg quality in IVF has now been observed in a range of other studies, including double-blind, placebo-controlled trials.[39] These studies report that supplementing with melatonin results in a higher number of good-quality eggs and embryos, or a higher pregnancy rate after IVF, or both. The benefits are often particularly clear for women undergoing IVF who have had failed IVF cycles due to poor egg quality or diminished ovarian reserve.

## Melatonin and endometriosis

If you are undergoing IVF in order to circumvent fertility problems caused by endometriosis, melatonin may have added benefits beyond supporting egg quality. A randomized, double-blind, placebo-controlled study found that when women with endometriosis supplemented with a relatively high dose of melatonin (10 mg) for eight weeks, there was almost a 40 percent reduction in pain. Melatonin also improved sleep quality and signficantly reduced the need for pain medication.[40] Animal studies have also found that melatonin can help shrink endometriosis lesions.[41]

## Melatonin outside the IVF context

Traditionally, melatonin has only been regarded as a useful fertility supplement for women undergoing IVF. When this book was first published in 2014, I suggested that women trying to conceive naturally should probably not take melatonin, on the basis that melatonin may have a direct role in regulating the production of hormones that control the ovulation cycle.[42] As a result, it is possible that a melatonin supplement could therefore disrupt the natural hormone balance and interfere with ovulation.

This is not such a concern in the context of IVF because large doses of hormones are given to artificially regulate the cycle, and ovulation does not need to be carefully orchestrated by natural hormone levels. For women about to go through an IVF cycle, melatonin is so beneficial for egg quality that any minor effects on hormones are seen as irrelevant. For women trying to conceive naturally, the reverse may be true, and disrupting ovulation may be too high a price to pay for the antioxidant benefits of melatonin.

Yet new research indicates that there is one exception where melatonin may be helpful for certain women trying to conceive naturally. Specifically, melatonin may have a beneficial effect on the hormones that regulate ovulation in women with PCOS. In 2018, researchers tried giving melatonin to 40 women with PCOS for six months.[43] It turns out that melatonin was able to partially correct the hormonal abnormalities that are characteristic of PCOS. The practical result was that 95 percent of the women experienced a normalization in menstrual cycles. This would be expected to have a profound benefit for fertility in those with PCOS.

The researchers commented that the way in which melatonin helped PCOS seemed to be unrelated to insulin, so it may complement other insulin-focused strategies to combat PCOS, such as supplementing with myo-inositol (discussed in the next chapter). Indeed, a separate study indicated that the combined effect of melatonin and myo-inositol in women with PCOS was greater than either alone, with a synergistic benefit for egg and embryo quality.[44]

## Adding a melatonin supplement

Fertility clinics that stay abreast of scientific research now routinely recommend melatonin supplements for women preparing for IVF cycles, particularly when poor egg quality is a concern.

The typical dose is 3 milligrams per day, taken shortly before bed. In the United States, melatonin is available over the counter in supplement form and the particular brand or formulation is not critical. In the United Kingdom, you will need a prescription.

The timing of when to start a melatonin supplement before IVF is still an open issue. Traditionally, doctors have advised patients to start taking it a few weeks before egg retrieval, or when injectable medications begin. There is evidence that even just this short time is beneficial—improving fertilization rates and the proportion of good-quality embryos.[45]

Yet there may be value in starting earlier. In a 2017 double-blind study, it was started on day 5 of the cycle before the IVF cycle.[46] In that study, the effect on egg quality was particularly pronounced. The women taking melatonin were twice as likely to have top-quality embryos compared to those in the placebo group. (The study was too small to show any effect on pregnancy rate though.)

Given this study, and what we know about egg development, it likely makes sense to take melatonin for at least one month before egg retrieval. Like most other egg-quality supplements, clinics typically advise patients to stop taking melatonin the day before egg retrieval.

Melatonin supplements may cause daytime drowsiness, dizziness, and irritability, and may worsen depression. If side effects bother you, switching to a smaller dose is likely to help.

If you are located outside the United States, one alternative to getting a prescription for a melatonin supplement is to buy tart cherry juice concentrate or a tart cherry juice supplement. This particular type of cherry naturally contains a small amount of melatonin, along with other beneficial antioxidants.

## Other Fertility-Boosting Antioxidants

If you are trying to conceive without IVF and therefore melatonin is not the right supplement for you, alternative antioxidant supplements may have similar benefits. Although these other antioxidants have not been studied as extensively, it is worth considering adding one of them to your supplement regimen. These other antioxidants can also be used in conjunction with melatonin if you are preparing for IVF and are particularly concerned about your egg quality.

## Vitamin E

Vitamin E is a fat-soluble antioxidant found in nuts, seeds, and oil. Preliminary research in animals and humans now suggests that vitamin E could have a beneficial effect on egg quality.[47] One of the most interesting examples is a human study that compared the ability of vitamin E and melatonin to reduce free radical damage in ovarian follicles. The researchers found that both supplements were effective, although a 200-times higher dose of vitamin E was required for the same level of protection against free radicals.[48] That is, 600 mg of vitamin E had a similar effect to 3 mg of melatonin.

This study used a high dose of vitamin E—about double the recommended maximum daily dose. To explain this in practical terms, vitamin E supplements are often labeled with "IU" for International Units, and 600 mg is equivalent to 900 IU. A typical prenatal multivitamin will contain 30–60 IU, while a typical vitamin E supplement will contain 400 IU.

Although vitamin E is generally regarded as very safe, the European Food Safety Authority has indicated that adults should not take more than 300 mg daily,[49] which is equivalent to 450 IU.[50] (That is because very high doses may slightly increase overall mortality in the long term, likely by way of a very minor increase in bleeding risk.)

The Colorado Center for Reproductive Medicine (CCRM), arguably the top IVF clinic in the United States, recommends that women preparing for IVF take 200 IU of vitamin E because "studies [suggest] that 400 IU may not be as good for overall health."[51] CCRM also warns that vitamin E should not be used by people who are taking aspirin, because it adds to the anticlotting effect of aspirin.

While a vitamin E supplement alone may not be enough to dramatically improve egg quality, every small incremental improvement in egg quality helps.

A study published in 2014 by Dr. Elizabeth Ruder and other researchers at the University of Pittsburgh, Emory University, and Dartmouth Medical Center adds further support to the view that vitamin E supplements are particularly useful for women with unexplained infertility.[52] The study involved over four hundred women with unexplained infertility who were trying to conceive through IUI and IVF. The researchers found that in the women who were over age 35, greater intake of vitamin E through supplements was linked to a shorter time to pregnancy.

Although further research is needed, experts now believe that vitamin E may compensate for some of the decline in antioxidants that naturally occurs as women age.[53] If you decide to take a vitamin E supplement in addition to the small amount of vitamin E in your prenatal multivitamin, it is best to err on the side of caution and look for one that contains no more than 200 IU.

As will be discussed in chapter 11, vitamin E also appears to be helpful for supporting the development of the uterine lining, in preparation for embryo transfer. As a result, there is likely an advantage in continuing to take vitamin E after egg retrieval, right up until the time of embryo transfer.

## Vitamin C

Vitamin C is a water-soluble antioxidant naturally found in large amounts in ovarian follicles.[54] In older mice, both vitamins C and E were found to prevent at least some of the age-related decline in ovarian function.[55] A vitamin C derivative also improved the quality of pig embryos in a lab study. In human studies, however, there is still limited evidence that taking additional vitamin C improves female fertility.

One of the few studies to date showing positive results from the use of vitamin C supplements is the same 2014 study described above in the context of vitamin E. In addition to investigating the value of vitamin E supplements, the study also explored whether vitamin C supplements were helpful to women with unexplained infertility.

The researchers found that at least for women of a healthy weight and women under the age of 35, increased vitamin C intake from supplements was associated with a shorter time to pregnancy.[56] This does not mean that vitamin C is thought to be less helpful to older or overweight women, but rather the effect was not seen in the study because the dose may have been too low for these groups. The researchers explained that in the overweight women, and most women in the older age bracket, their vitamin C intake was likely not sufficient to make up for their already high levels of oxidation.

In 2018, researchers conducted a randomized controlled trial of vitamin C supplements for women with endometriosis who were trying to conceive through IVF.[57] The women were randomized to receive either no additional supplement or 1000 mg of vitamin C per day for two months before the IVF cycle. Those in the vitamin C group ended up with a significantly higher number of good-quality embryos. The women taking vitamin C also had a slightly higher chance of pregnancy, although the study was too small to show statistical significance for this outcome.

If you choose to add a vitamin C supplement, the typical dose is 500 mg per day, or 1000 mg per day for those with endometriosis.

## Alpha-Lipoic Acid

Alpha-lipoic acid is another supplement that has well-established antioxidant properties and may therefore benefit egg quality.[58] It is naturally produced in the body and has the rare ability to act as both a water-soluble and fat-soluble antioxidant.[59] By contrast, vitamin C is water soluble and vitamin E is fat soluble, so those antioxidants have more limited reach.

Alpha-lipoic acid is also a promising supplement because it is found naturally in mitochondria, where it assists in energy production.[60] Animal studies have found that alpha-lipoic acid can protect mitochondria from the effects of aging.[61] When people take alpha-lipoic acid supplements, the total antioxidant level in the bloodstream increases significantly, and there is an increase in the activity of antioxidant enzymes.[62]

There is also some evidence that alpha-lipoic acid improves fertility. For example, laboratory studies have found that this antioxidant can improve egg maturation and embryo viability.[63]

As discussed in chapter 14, this antioxidant improves sperm quality too. When men took 600 mg of alpha-lipoic acid each day for 12 weeks in a randomized, double-blind, placebo-controlled study, there was a significant improvement in the total sperm count, sperm concentration, and motility levels.[64]

Alpha-lipoic acid is a particularly beneficial antioxidant because it helps recycle CoQ10, vitamin C, and vitamin E back into their active antioxidant form. Alpha-lipoic acid also helps increase the level of another critical antioxidant called glutathione.

In women, the benefit of alpha-lipoic acid for fertility is particularly clear for those with PCOS. Researchers have found, for example, that the combination of alpha-lipoic acid and myo-inositol is superior to myo-inositol alone, resulting in a higher number of good-quality embryos after IVF.[65]

In a separate study published in 2017, it was reported that when women with PCOS took the combination of alpha-lipoic acid and myo-inositol for six months, the hormonal abnormalities that are characteristic of PCOS normalized.[66] Another study found that women with PCOS who took 600 mg twice a day for 16 weeks had improved insulin sensitivity and began ovulating normally.[67]

Even though most of the human studies of alpha lipoic acid in the fertility context have focused on sperm quality or PCOS, the way in which this molecule works suggests it is helpful across the board, whenever egg quality is an issue. That is because it is a powerful antioxidant that also supports energy production in the mitochondria.

Alpha-lipoic acid also reduces inflammation and may therefore have even greater benefit for those with endometriosis or recurrent miscarriage.[68] Research indicates that inflammation may be one of the key ways in which endometriosis causes infertility. New studies have also found that inflammation may be a major contributor to unexplained miscarriage. (This topic will be discussed further in the chapter on diet.)

## Safety and side effects of alpha-lipoic acid

In clinical trials of alpha-lipoic acid, no significant side effects have been reported. The most common side effect is nausea, but even this is rare at doses of 600 mg per day.[69]

It has been suggested that alpha-lipoic acid may lower thyroid hormones,[70] so if you have thyroid problems, you should not take this supplement before discussing it with your doctor. Alpha-lipoic acid may also improve blood sugar levels in diabetics,[71] so if you have diabetes you should be carefully monitored when you start taking this supplement. Ultimately, your doctor may be able to decrease the dose of your diabetes medication.

## Dosage and form of alpha-lipoic acid

The clinical studies show that alpha-lipoic acid is typically effective at a dose of 400–600 milligrams per day (although some have used 1200 milligrams per day for PCOS). If you choose a supplement that is in the form of R-alpha lipoic acid, it is likely sufficient to take 200–300 milligrams per day. That is because R-alpha lipoic acid is the more biologically active form that is naturally made in the body.[72]

If a supplement does not specify the R-form, it is likely a 50 percent mixture of R-alpha lipoic acid and its mirror image molecule, which is less effective. Choosing the R-form of alpha-lipoic acid allows you to use a lower dose, which reduces the stomach discomfort that can sometimes occur with this supplement.

Alpha-lipoic acid may also be better absorbed on an empty stomach, so the standard advice is to take it 30 minutes before or two hours after eating.[73] Nevertheless, if taking it on an empty stomach is inconvenient or causes nausea or heartburn, taking the supplement with meals will only reduce the amount you absorb by about 20–30 percent.

For those with a sensitive stomach, the best option is to take 100 mg R-alpha lipoic acid (such as Pure Encapsulations R-lipoic acid) two or three times per day with meals. Others can take 200 or 300 mg of R-alpha lipoic acid all at once on an empty stomach, once per day.

## N-Acetylcysteine

Another antioxidant that may benefit egg quality and fertility is called N-acetylcysteine. This amino acid derivative acts as an antioxidant and also boosts the activity of glutathione, another critical antioxidant inside cells.[74] It is commonly used as an antidote to poisoning from overdose of acetaminophen (also known as Tylenol or paracetamol).[75]

## N-acetylcysteine and PCOS

The clearest evidence demonstrating the ability of N-acetylcysteine to improve fertility comes from clinical trials in PCOS. There has now been a series of randomized, double-blind, placebo-controlled studies finding that in women with PCOS, supplementing with N-acetylcysteine restores ovulation, improves egg and embryo quality, increases the chance of pregnancy, and reduces miscarriage rates.[76] This has been seen in women trying to conceive naturally, those taking medications such as Clomid or letrozole, and those trying to conceive through IVF.

The difference that N-acetylcysteine makes is perhaps most dramatic in the women with PCOS who have been struggling with infertility the longest. In one clinical trial, women with PCOS who on average had suffered from infertility for more than four years took N-acetylcysteine and the ovulation-stimulating drug Clomid for five days. After treatment, 21 percent of the women taking N-acetylcysteine became pregnant, compared to 9 percent of women taking the placebo.[77]

## N-acetylcysteine beyond PCOS

Although the majority of studies so far have focused on PCOS, researchers believe it may also improve egg quality and fertility more generally. Specifically, by acting as an antioxidant, and supporting detoxification, it may counteract the effect of aging and oxidative stress on egg quality.

This was seen in a recent study where women were randomly assigned to take a placebo or N-acetylcysteine while preparing for IVF.[78] In the group taking the supplement, more eggs were retrieved and the pregnancy rate was much higher (74 percent versus 50 percent). There was also a much lower level of the toxin homocysteine in ovarian follicles.

If N-acetylcysteine can reduce homocysteine levels in ovarian follicles, that has wide implications for a range of causes of infertility. Homocysteine is incredibly damaging for developing eggs, because it damages mitochondria. One of the main ways in which folate boosts fertility is by detoxifying homocysteine. It is clearly helpful to have yet another tool to help with this important detoxification work and thereby support energy production in developing eggs.

N-acetylcysteine may therefore be particularly important for those with risk factors associated with high homocysteine levels, such as genetic variations in folate metabolism genes (including MTHFR), and those with premature ovarian failure, or a history of recurrent miscarriage.

## Preventing miscarriage with N-acetylcysteine

Just as we would expect from its ability to reduce inflammation and homocysteine, N-acetylcysteine does appear to reduce miscarriage risk.

This was seen when a group of women with unexplained recurrent miscarriage were given 600 mg per day along with folic acid, and the pregnancy outcomes compared to women taking folic acid alone. The combination of N-acetylcysteine and folic acid was associated with a very dramatic decrease in the chance of miscarriage. Ultimately, the women taking N-acetylcysteine were twice as likely to take a baby home.[79]

Other studies have also shown that N-acetylcysteine decreases the miscarriage rate by 60 percent in women with PCOS.[80]

## N-acetylcysteine and endometriosis

N-acetylcysteine may also be particularly helpful for those with endometriosis. In a recent laboratory study, researchers demonstrated that this antioxidant can help counteract the negative influence of endometriosis on egg quality.[81] In addition, a clinical study in Italy found that in women with endometriosis, taking N-acetylcysteine can actually reduce the pain and cysts associated with endometriosis.[82] After three months of treatment, one-third of the patients taking N-acetylcysteine showed such improvement that their surgery was cancelled. In the words of the study authors, "we can conclude that NAC actually represents a simple effective treatment for endometriosis, without side effects, and a suitable approach for women desiring a pregnancy."

## Safety and side effects of N-acetylcysteine

N-acetylcysteine is widely used by doctors for a variety of conditions,[83] but allergies and side effects sometimes occur. Rarely, allergic reactions have occurred after the use of high doses of intravenous N-acetylcysteine to treat painkiller overdose.[84] In some people, N-acetylcysteine also causes nausea, diarrhea, or abdominal pain. If these side effects bother you, it likely makes sense to stop the supplement and focus on the other antioxidants discussed in this chapter.

## Dosage of N-acetylcysteine

In clinical trials where N-acetylcysteine is taken for several months, the typical dose is 600 mg per day. In the PCOS studies, where N-acetylcysteine was only given for five days, the dose used was 1200 mg per day. From what we understand about egg quality and the time it takes for eggs to develop, it probably makes sense to take the lower dose for a longer period of time where possible.

## N-Acetylcysteine versus Acetyl-L-Carnitine

Acetyl-L-carnitine is another antioxidant molecule that is often confused with N-acetylcysteine, but they are entirely different molecules. The liver produces carnitine from the amino acid lysine. Some of this is then converted into acetyl-L-carnitine.

Carnitine (whether as L-carnitine or acetyl-L-carnitine) is often taken as a sports and weight loss supplement because it helps in the conversion of fat into cellular energy. Research shows that this supplement is also likely to benefit sperm quality, because it is an antioxidant that participates in energy production in the mitochondria. Yet the effect on egg quality is still quite uncertain.

In the context of female fertility, most of the research to date has focused on the L-carnitine form, specifically in the context of PCOS. Randomized clinical trials have found that in women with PCOS, L-carnitine supports weight loss, regulates insulin levels, restores ovulation, helps eggs develop to maturity, and improves pregnancy rates.[85] These studies fit together with the finding that L-carnitine levels are often significantly lower in women with PCOS.[86] If you have PCOS, L-carnitine is therefore one additional supplement to consider, typically at a dose of 3 grams per day.

For women without PCOS, there is not enough evidence at this stage to support the use of either L-carnitine or acetyl-L-carnitine. The majority of animal studies have found beneficial effects for female fertility, but others have reported the opposite.[87] A human study published in 2017 found a beneficial effect on embryo quality,[88] yet it is still too early to know for sure whether this supplement is beneficial for women. For men, the evidence is much stronger, as discussed in chapter 14.

## Conclusion

Many experts believe that oxidative stress is a major mechanism underlying ovarian aging.[89] To prevent oxidative damage to eggs, reactive oxygen molecules (such as free radicals) must be continuously kept in check by the eggs' natural antioxidants. But in women with age-related infertility, endometriosis, PCOS, or unexplained infertility, this natural antioxidant defense system may be compromised, creating a need for further antioxidants.

How many and which antioxidants you should add to your supplement regime depends on the particular fertility challenge you are facing, but it is reasonable to choose two or three antioxidants—ideally those that are most likely to help with your specific concern. The options are summarized in the list below, and specific examples of supplement regimes for various scenarios are provided in chapter 12.

- Melatonin
    - › Best for: IVF or PCOS
    - › Typical dose: 3 mg before bed
- Vitamin E
    - › Best for: unexplained or age-related infertility, prep for embryo transfer
    - › Typical dose: 200 IU vitamin E
- Vitamin C
    - › Best for: unexplained or age-related infertility, endometriosis
    - › Typical dose: 500–1000 mg

- Alpha-lipoic Acid

  › Best for: PCOS, age-related infertility, diminished ovarian reserve, autoimmunity, recurrent miscarriage, and endometriosis

  › Typical dose: 200–300 mg R-alpha lipoic acid (or 600 mg standard form)

- N-acetylcysteine

  › Best for: PCOS, age-related infertility, diminished ovarian reserve, endometriosis, MTHFR variants, and recurrent miscarriage

  › Typical dose: 600 mg

Antioxidants can typically be stopped shortly before egg retrieval (in the case of IVF), or when you get a positive pregnancy test. If you are trying to conceive by IVF, it may be worthwhile continuing vitamin E until the time of embryo transfer, as will be covered in chapter 11.

# CHAPTER 8

# Restoring Ovulation with Myo-Inositol

*"Sometimes the questions are compli-cated and the answers are simple."*

— DR. SEUSS

## Recommended for
## Intermediate and Advanced Fertility Plans

MYO-INOSITOL IS PARTICULARLY helpful for restoring ovulation and improving egg quality in women with PCOS or insulin resistance. In some cases, it may also be helpful even if you do not have PCOS. Specifically, myo-inositol is worth considering if you have had a previous IVF cycle in which many eggs were immature, you have a history of unexplained recurrent miscarriage, or you are not ovulating regularly.

## Not recommended for

Many studies have shown that myo-inositol is very safe, with few or no side effects. Myo-inositol should, however, be used with caution if you have schizophrenia or bipolar disorder because there is a theoretical risk of exacerbating manic episodes.[1]

### What is Myo-Inositol?

Myo-inositol is a type of sugar molecule naturally found in a variety of foods, such as fruits, vegetables, grains, and nuts. It is generally regarded as a type of B vitamin (vitamin B8), but it is not truly an essential vitamin, because the body can produce it from glucose. Myo-inositol plays a variety of roles in the body, including acting as a key building block for signaling molecules.

Myo-inositol has recently become a widely recommended fertility supplement, yet the story of myo-inositol's role in egg quality began many years ago. In 2002, Dr. Tony Chiu and a group of researchers in Hong Kong published the results of the first study to directly link myo-inositol to egg and embryo quality.[2] They tracked the levels of myo-inositol inside each ovarian follicle in 53 women undergoing IVF and then compared the amount of myo-inositol in each follicle to the quality of the egg inside and whether it later fertilized.

The results were unambiguous. Higher levels of myo-inositol were found in ovarian follicles containing mature eggs that later successfully fertilized. In addition, there was a clear link between higher myo-inositol levels in follicles and higher-quality embryos.

Dr. Chiu was inspired to investigate myo-inositol by much earlier research showing that this compound is a precursor to important signaling molecules called inositol phospho-lipids. These signaling molecules communicate messages and thereby regulate a wide range of biological activities inside cells, including in developing eggs.

The link between myo-inositol and egg quality raised an intriguing possibility to researchers: Perhaps adding extra myo-inositol in the form of a supplement could improve the chances of success in IVF. It took many years to test that hypothesis, but there is now solid evidence that myo-inositol supplements can improve fertility, at least in women with PCOS or insulin resistance (as will be discussed further below).

## What If You Don't Have PCOS?

For women without PCOS or insulin resistance, the value of myo-inositol is still uncertain. To date, there has only been a small number of studies of women without PCOS and the results have not been hugely impressive.[3] In the first of these studies, doctors gave myo-inositol to women without PCOS for three months before an IVF cycle. Myo-inositol actually seemed to reduce the number of mature eggs and embryos. While the implantation rate and pregnancy rates were slightly higher in the myo-inositol group compared to the group given a placebo, the study was too small to test whether this difference was real or occurred by chance.

In a similar study, this time involving women without PCOS who were categorized as "poor responders" after previous failed IVF cycles, myo-inositol actually significantly increased the number of mature eggs obtained.[4] There was also a small increase in the number of good-quality embryos, the implantation rate, and the pregnancy rate in the women who had taken myo-inositol.

This limited evidence probably does not justify adding this supplement under ordinary circumstances, but based on the evidence discussed below in the context of PCOS, myo-inositol may be worth considering if

- in previous IVF cycles, many eggs were immature.
- you have insulin resistance.
- you have irregular or long cycles (more than 30 days).
- you have hormonal disruptions that are commonly associated with PCOS (such as high testosterone or high AMH).

As will be discussed further below, myo-inositol may also play a role in preventing miscarriage in some cases.

### Myo-inositol and PCOS

To understand why myo-inositol is so beneficial in PCOS, we need to go back to the underlying cause of the hormonal imbalances in this condition. Doctors have known for more than 30 years that PCOS is associated with high insulin levels, even in women of a healthy weight.[5] High insulin levels appear to have a direct role in causing infertility in PCOS by increasing levels of hormones such as testosterone in the ovaries.[6]

Based on this understanding, PCOS has been treated with various drugs that make the body more responsive to insulin. These drugs aim to make cells more sensitive to insulin's message to take up glucose from the bloodstream, thereby better controlling blood glucose levels and lowering insulin levels. One example is metformin, which has been widely studied for improving blood sugar control in PCOS and diabetes.[7]

The theory of using metformin to improve fertility in PCOS is that by returning insulin levels to normal, we could also rebalance reproductive hormones and restore ovulation. Metformin, however, has some significant side effects, such as nausea and vomiting,[8] and it is not clear how well it works.

Against this background, scientists began looking for alternatives for improving insulin function in women with PCOS, with the goal of ultimately improving fertility. This is where the story returns to myo-inositol. It was already known that some molecules in the inositol family are involved in insulin function and sugar metabolism. It was also known that myo-inositol may be depleted in PCOS. The final piece of the puzzle was Dr. Chiu's experiments showing higher levels of myo-inositol in follicles associated with good-quality eggs.

Researchers now believe that a defect in the processing of molecules in the inositol family may contribute to insulin resistance in PCOS.[9] A myo-inositol supplement may circumvent this problem to both rebalance insulin and restore the necessary levels of myo-inositol in developing eggs.[10]

Many studies have now consistently shown that taking a myo-inositol supplement is indeed beneficial in women with PCOS. In one of the first studies, published in 2007, 25 women with PCOS took a myo-inositol supplement for six months. Before the study began, all these women had experienced at least one year of infertility and fewer than six menstrual cycles per year, and it had been determined that the most likely cause of their infertility was ovulation dysfunction. Over the course of the six months taking myo-inositol, 72 percent of these women began ovulating normally again.[11] More than half of these women then became pregnant.

Similar results were reached in several later studies, [12] including a study in which both doctor and patient were blind as to whether a particular patient was assigned to myo-inositol or a placebo, minimizing the possibility of bias and the placebo effect.[13] The results were stark: In women receiving myo-inositol, nearly 70 percent ovulated compared to just 21 percent ovulating after taking the placebo.

All these studies showing restored ovulation and improved chances of conceiving naturally are just one part of the story. At a more granular level, IVF cycles have also allowed doctors to directly observe the positive impact of myo-inositol on egg and embryo quality in women with PCOS.

In the first IVF study showing this positive impact, women were given myo-inositol starting on the day of the IVF medications. Myo-inositol was found to increase the proportion of mature eggs retrieved and decrease the number of immature and degenerated eggs, compared to women not receiving myo-inositol.[14] In addition, fewer cycles were canceled because of concern about overstimulating the ovaries.

When the myo-inositol supplement was started earlier, it had an even greater impact on IVF outcomes in women with PCOS.[15] In a double-blind trial, doctors gave women 2 grams of myo-inositol plus folic acid twice a day for three months and gave a second group folic acid alone. When the women underwent IVF, those who had been taking myo-inositol had more mature follicles, more eggs retrieved, and fewer imma-ture eggs retrieved compared to women taking folic acid alone. Interestingly, this study also found a much higher pro-portion of top-quality embryos in women taking myo-ino-sitol: 68 percent versus 29 percent in the women taking only folic acid.

In short, myo-inositol seems to improve egg development and embryo quality in women with PCOS, along with lowering insulin and improving blood sugar control. And it is not just women with poor insulin sensitivity who can benefit. A study conducted in Italy and published in 2011 found that even in PCOS patients having a normal insulin response, myo-inositol treatment improved egg and embryo quality during IVF.[16]

## PCOS and gestational diabetes

If you have PCOS, taking myo-inositol could have another added benefit: reducing your risk of gestational diabetes. This condition, which involves high blood sugar levels during preg-nancy, is much more common in women with PCOS.

In 2012, researchers found that women with PCOS taking a myo-inositol supplement during their pregnancy had a much lower risk of gestational diabetes: just 17 percent compared to 54 percent in women not taking the supplement.[17] Several other clinical trials have now reported similar positive results. In 2015, the Cochrane Organization reviewed the trials avail-able at that time and concluded that myo-inositol does show a potential benefit for reducing the incidence of gestational dia-betes. If you have PCOS, or other risk factors for gestational diabetes, you should therefore ask your doctor whether to continue taking myo-inositol during pregnancy.

## Myo-inositol and miscarriage

Myo-inositol may also have a role to play in preventing miscarriage in women with recurrent pregnancy loss. Studies have found a much higher rate of insulin resistance in women with a history of multiple miscarriages.[18] In one study, insulin resistance was two to three times more common in this group.[19]

In theory, if insulin resistance contributes to the risk of miscarriage, a supplement that reverses insulin resistance, such as myo-inositol, could be beneficial. To determine if this may be helpful in your case, you can ask your doctor for a glucose tolerance test, where blood glucose is measured while fasting and then two hours after drinking a sugar solution. If you are found to have insulin resistance, it could theoretically be helpful to add a myo-inositol supplement to reduce your miscarriage risk.

## Safety, Side Effects, and Dose

Myo-inositol has been described as very safe, with only high doses of 12 g per day causing mild gastrointestinal symptoms such as nausea.[20] The typical recommended dose, shown to be effective in clinical studies, is 4 g per day, divided into two doses: half in the morning and half at night. This is similar to the amount of myo-inositol naturally produced in the body each day. Ideally, myo-inositol should be taken for at least three months before IVF. Talk to your doctor about when to stop the supplement. Many doctors recommend that women with PCOS continue myo-inositol through pregnancy to prevent gestational diabetes.

## What About D-Chiro Inositol?

A similar-sounding and related compound, D-chiro inositol, is often used by women with PCOS in the hope of improving their fertility, but in large doses it may have just the opposite effect: reducing the number and quality of eggs.[21] This negative effect is unfortunately not widely known. The early studies showing a possible benefit of D-chiro inositol have overshadowed the more recent studies showing that the supplement simply does not work or may do more harm than good.[22] As just one example, one study found that women with PCOS who were given D-chiro inositol rather than a placebo had fewer eggs and fewer good-quality embryos.[23]

Researchers are now beginning to understand why D-chiro inositol is so unhelpful in PCOS. In the body, an enzyme converts a small proportion of myo-inositol to D-chiro inositol to maintain the proper ratio for different parts of the body. In the liver and muscles, the normal ratio is approximately 40:1, with 40 parts myo-inositol to 1 part D-chiro inositol. In the ovaries, the normal proportion of myo-inositol is even greater, with a ratio of approximately 100:1.

The two closely related molecules actually have distinct jobs to do in the ovaries. Myo-inositol supports the function of follicle-stimulating hormone (FSH), while D-chiro inositol supports testosterone production.[24] It appears that PCOS may involve overactive conversion of myo-inositol into D-chiro inositol, depleting normal levels of myo-inositol and causing excess testosterone production.[25] This could in turn cause poor egg quality, which would explain why myo-inositol could improve egg quality, while supplementing with large amounts of D-chiro inositol could simply make the problem worse.

Some of the popular myo-inositol supplements marketed for fertility purposes, such as Ovasitol, include a small amount of D-chiro inositol. The idea behind this combination is mimicking the 40:1 ratio of myo-inositol to D-chiro inositol that is naturally found in the body. This combination supplement has been shown to improve metabolic function and ovulation in women with PCOS,[26] but there is currently a much larger body of evidence supporting the use of myo-inositol alone.

## Conclusion

Myo-inositol is now routinely recommended for women with PCOS because it appears to restore normal ovulation, improve egg quality, and prevent gestational diabetes. If you have PCOS, taking a daily myo-inositol supplement for several weeks or months could be incredibly helpful. Myo-inositol may also improve fertility in women who do not ovulate or who have insulin resistance. There is a possibility that myo-inositol could also reduce miscarriage risk linked to insulin resistance, but further research is needed.

# CHAPTER 9

# DHEA for Diminished Ovarian Reserve

*"Don't be discouraged. It's often the last key in the bunch that opens the lock."*
— UNKNOWN

## Recommended for:
## Advanced Plan

D HEA IS NOW widely recommended by fertility clinics for women with diminished ovarian reserve or age-related infertility who are preparing for IVF.[1] The science supporting the use of DHEA is controversial, but research suggests that it may improve egg numbers and quality. DHEA may also reduce miscarriage risk by increasing the proportion of chromosomally normal eggs.

## Not recommended for:

Even though DHEA is sold over the counter as a nutritional supplement, it is actually a hormone, so you should talk to your fertility specialist before taking it. It can interact with some medications and is generally not recommended for those with PCOS or a history of hormone-sensitive cancer. It has not been studied extensively in women with endometriosis.

## An Introduction to DHEA

The story of DHEA started with one woman, a determined patient at an IVF clinic in New York who was over 40 and searching for anything that could improve her odds. In her own research, she uncovered a scientific article about DHEA improving egg numbers in IVF and started taking the supplement. The results were so astounding that her clinic quickly became pioneers in the use of DHEA to improve IVF outcomes.

Several years later, DHEA is now routinely recommended for certain IVF patients to increase the number and quality of eggs and embryos. According to Dr. Norbert Gleicher, a leading fertility specialist, "DHEA is in the process of revolutionizing infertility care for older women and for younger women with premature aging ovaries."[2]

## What Is DHEA?

DHEA stands for dehydroepiandrosterone. It is a hormone precursor produced by the adrenals and ovaries. DHEA is critical for early development of ovarian follicles. If for any reason the adrenals are not producing enough DHEA, fewer eggs will go through the early stages of development at any given time, resulting in a lower follicle count on ultrasound and hormone levels that are typically indicative of low ovarian reserve or ovarian aging (such as low AMH).

Levels of DHEA typically decline with age, and this is thought to be one possible cause of age-related infertility.[3] DHEA levels may also be low in younger women with autoimmune conditions, such as thyroid disease, rheumatoid arthritis, or antibodies that attack the adrenal glands. Autoimmunity is now understood to be a common cause of premature ovarian insufficiency in young women.[4] If testing shows that your DHEA levels are low, correcting this deficiency can make a dramatic difference to your fertility—potentially increasing both the number and quality of eggs available for retrieval in IVF.

## The Discovery of DHEA Boosting Fertility

The pioneers in the use of DHEA to increase fertility are the reproductive endocrinologists at the Center for Human Reproduction (CHR), a large IVF clinic in New York with a surprisingly high success rate in older patients with low ovarian reserve. Their work on DHEA began with a single patient, a 43-year-old woman scouring the medical literature for anything that could help improve her egg numbers.

In her first IVF cycle, before taking DHEA, she produced just a single egg and embryo, and her doctors discouraged further attempts at IVF using her own eggs. Determined to have a child with her own eggs, she began her own search of the scientific literature for anything that could help.

During this research, she stumbled upon a publication from researchers at Baylor University suggesting a possible benefit of DHEA in IVF cycles.[5] The Baylor study described an increase in egg numbers in five women taking DHEA for two months, but it received very little attention until it was rediscovered and put to the test several years later by this individual patient in New York.

After reading the Baylor paper, she began taking DHEA supplements, unbeknownst to her doctors. In her second IVF cycle, she produced three eggs and embryos.

Amazingly, as she continued taking DHEA, her egg and embryo numbers progressively increased.[6] She explains, "I was beginning to realize I was onto something."[7] Her doctors report being astonished because at her age she should have been getting worse, not better.[8] She ultimately produced 16 embryos in her ninth IVF cycle.[9]

This continuous improvement in egg numbers suggested that the beneficial effects of DHEA were cumulative. It is now understood that this longer-term effect is because DHEA acts on very early–stage follicles that are several months away from ovulation.

By 2011, just six years after the first extraordinary results with DHEA, a substantial number of IVF clinics worldwide began recommending DHEA supplements for women with diminished ovarian reserve.[10] Now, as further clinical evidence has emerged, even more clinics have adopted this strategy for improving IVF outcomes.

## Who Should Consider Taking DHEA?

Most of the research on DHEA has focused on women with a condition called "diminished ovarian reserve." Often the cause is age. As women reach their mid- to late thirties, the pool of follicles recruited each month to begin maturing shrinks in number. As a result, the number of eggs that can be stimulated by medication and then retrieved in an IVF cycle declines. This becomes a limiting factor to IVF success rates for women in their late thirties and forties, and women over 40 are universally assumed to have diminished ovarian reserve.

Diminished ovarian reserve also sometimes affects much younger women, in which case the term "premature ovarian aging" or "premature ovarian insufficiency" is sometimes used. In younger women, the condition is often diagnosed by measuring the level of a hormone called AMH, which reflects the number of follicles in very early stages of maturing. Doctors also perform an ultrasound to count the number of early stage follicles. If you have a low AMH or a low follicle count (or both), you may be diagnosed with diminished ovarian reserve.

Women with diminished ovarian reserve often overlap with the group of patients called "poor responders," in which the ovaries do not respond as expected to stimulation medication in an IVF cycle, and very few mature eggs are retrieved.

Poor responders and women with diminished ovarian reserve or premature ovarian aging typically have very low success rates in IVF, and cycles are often canceled because there are not enough eggs to retrieve. Research on DHEA has focused on these particular patients because this type of infertility is incredibly difficult to treat, and DHEA appears to get at the core of the problem by increasing the number of eggs produced in an IVF cycle.

Based on current research, fertility specialists typically only recommend DHEA if you have been diagnosed with diminished ovarian reserve, you are over the age of 40 (some clinics say 35) or have had an IVF cycle that produced very few eggs. If you fall into one of these groups, DHEA may significantly improve your chance of conceiving, as described in the research that follows.

## The Clinical Studies on DHEA

After witnessing extraordinary results in their first patient taking DHEA, the fertility specialists at CHR in New York began an initial study to find out whether DHEA could offer the same benefit to other women with diminished ovarian reserve who had little hope of producing enough eggs for a successful IVF cycle.

The group gave DHEA supplements to 25 patients with diminished ovarian reserve who were planning IVF. At the end of the IVF cycle, the resulting egg and embryo numbers were compared to each woman's previous IVF cycle without DHEA.[11] The results were impressive, showing increases in egg and embryo numbers along with improved egg quality.

This initial study was then followed up with a larger study in which women with diminished ovarian reserve were given DHEA for four months and the IVF outcomes compared to controls. In this study, the beneficial effects of DHEA on egg and embryos were again clearly apparent and translated into much higher pregnancy rates. Specifically, 28 percent of DHEA-treated women became pregnant, compared to just 10 percent of controls.[12]

Since that time, many other studies have confirmed that women with diminished ovarian reserve taking DHEA supplements before IVF have a much higher chance of becoming pregnant. This has been seen in numerous randomized, controlled studies, in which women preparing for IVF are randomly assigned to take DHEA or not for two to four months before IVF.[13]

In 2015, the independent Cochrane organization conducted a review of these studies and reached the following conclusion:

"We included 17 [randomized controlled trials] with a total of 1496 participants. Apart from two trials, the trial participants were women identified as 'poor responders' to standard IVF protocols. The included trials compared either testosterone or DHEA treatment with placebo or no treatment. When DHEA was compared with placebo or no treatment, pre-treatment with DHEA was associated with higher rates of live birth or ongoing pregnancy... The overall quality of the evidence was moderate."

In the years since that review, the evidence has only strengthened. A controlled trial published in 2016, for example, found that women receiving DHEA before IVF had a much higher pregnancy rate than the controls (33 percent versus 16 percent).[14] A 2018 study showed similar results.[15]

When the current data from all the highest quality studies is pooled together and subject to thorough statistical analysis (a so-called "meta-analysis"), there is a clear and consistent answer: in poor responders, DHEA treatment before IVF results in a significantly higher likelihood of pregnancy.[16]

## DHEA Outside the IVF Context

DHEA also appears to boost pregnancy chances for those trying to conceive naturally or through IUI. In the case of IUI, fertility specialists in Toronto reported positive results of treating women with DHEA for several months before insemination, in conjunction with Clomid treatment. Compared to controls, DHEA-treated women showed higher follicle counts and improved pregnancy rates, with 29.8 percent conceiving versus 8.7 percent in the nontreated group, and a live birth rate of 21.3 percent versus 6.5 percent.[17]

Researchers have also reported surprising numbers of naturally conceived pregnancies in women taking DHEA while waiting for IVF. A group of doctors in Italy were so intrigued by the number of women conceiving spontaneously while taking DHEA that they decided to conduct a study to specifically investigate this phenomenon. In a paper published in 2013, the doctors reported that from a group of 39 younger "poor responders" taking DHEA for three months before starting IVF, 10 of these women became pregnant naturally before the IVF cycle began.[18]

The same phenomenon was also seen in women over 40, with 21 percent conceiving while taking DHEA in preparation for IVF, compared to just 4 percent of women in the control group. This is an extraordinary finding that requires further confirmation, but it is in line with anecdotal reports from several other fertility clinics.[19] If correct, these results indicate that DHEA may improve fertility enough for some women with diminished ovarian reserve to conceive even without IVF.[20]

## DHEA and miscarriage

Although the evidence in this regard is still somewhat uncertain, it appears that DHEA may also reduce chromosomal abnormalities in eggs and thereby help prevent miscarriages. A study of IVF patients in two independent fertility clinics in New York and Toronto reported a surprisingly low miscarriage rate in women taking DHEA.[21] In this study, pregnancy loss was reduced by 50–80 percent in comparison to national US IVF pregnancy rates, bringing the miscarriage rate down to just 15 percent of pregnancies.

This low miscarriage rate is all the more surprising since women with diminished ovarian reserve are known to have much higher miscarriage rates than women with other causes of infertility.[22] After treatment with DHEA, the miscarriage rate dropped to the normal level seen in women without diminished ovarian reserve.[23]

Miscarriage rates are thought to be so high in women with diminished ovarian reserve because the vast majority of eggs are chromosomally abnormal (aneuploid). The CHR group noted that DHEA appears to decrease miscarriage rates to a degree that cannot be explained without a significant reduction of chromosomal abnormalities.[24] In other words, it would be mathematically impossible to reduce miscarriage rates to just 15 percent without reducing aneuploidy rates.

The CHR group then set out to delve into that question a little further by looking at data from women who underwent IVF and had their embryos screened for chromosomal abnormalities. Within this patient population, the researchers identified a group of women with diminished ovarian reserve treated with DHEA and matched them to a control group that did not receive DHEA treatment.

Because diminished ovarian reserve is associated with very high levels of aneuploidy, one would expect much higher rates of aneuploidy in the diminished ovarian reserve group than in controls, but instead the reverse happened. In the control group, 61 percent of embryos were chromosomally abnormal, whereas only 38 percent of embryos from DHEA-treated women with diminished ovarian reserve were chromosomally abnormal.[25] This very promising result suggests that DHEA may indeed reduce the rate of chromosomal abnormalities and therefore reduce the risk of miscarriage.

A reduction in miscarriage rates has not been seen in every study on DHEA, but when researchers recently looked at all the data from the controlled trials of DHEA for poor responders undergoing IVF, they did find a general trend of lower miscarriage rates in those women who took DHEA.[26]

If true, this has wide implications for the way we understand egg quality and age-related infertility. It suggests that the increase in chromosomal abnormalities with age and diminished ovarian reserve are not a foregone conclusion; external factors such as hormones can, to some extent, correct the problem.

## How Does DHEA Work?

DHEA likely plays such an important role in egg development because it is necessary for the production of hormones such as testosterone. Although normally considered a male hormone, testosterone actually performs important work in the ovaries too. It binds to androgen receptors on the surface of ovarian cells and encourages more early stage follicles to develop each month. When testosterone is low, this can cause a low follicle count and low AMH. Supplementing with DHEA likely improves fertility in part by replenishing testosterone levels, to support the earliest phase of egg development.

So why not directly supplement with testosterone? This question was recently answered by Dr. Gleicher, Dr. Barad, and Dr. Kushnir from The Center for Human Reproduction:

"Since androgen levels vary in different organs, DHEA supplementation allows each organ, ovaries included, to draw organ-specific amounts of precursor to reach desirable testosterone levels. Direct administration of testosterone in approximately 15% of cases becomes necessary because older women in particular do not convert DHEA well to testosterone. However, in contrast to DHEA, testosterone floods all organs uniformly, overexposing some and underexposing others. Side effects with direct testosterone administration, therefore, are more pronounced."

By supporting testosterone production when and where it is needed, DHEA promotes the growth of very early–stage follicles—those follicles a couple of months away from ovulation.[27] It either increases the number of follicles that enter the early phase of maturing at any given time, or increases the proportion that survive this phase. Either way, the net result is a higher number of eggs available for IVF.[28]

Although not yet clearly established, DHEA may also improve the quality of those eggs, by reducing the rate of chromosomal abnormalities.[29] This outcome has only been reported in one study so far, but it fits with early research that found a link between chromosomal errors in eggs and lower levels of DHEA and testosterone in ovarian follicles.[30]

## The Current State of Play on DHEA

By some estimates, one-third of IVF clinics are now recommending DHEA to their patients with diminished ovarian reserve. Given the consistency of the data showing that DHEA increases the chance of pregnancy, how do we explain the other two-thirds of clinics who are not yet recommending DHEA?

It likely comes down to doctors either not staying up to date with the current research or being extremely conservative and waiting for the perfect large clinical trial that provides incontrovertible proof. Although we now have an array of randomized and placebo-controlled clinical trials showing clear benefits from DHEA, many of these studies are not "double-blind" studies, meaning that the patients know whether they have been randomly assigned to the DHEA group or the control group. Theoretically, this means we cannot rule out a placebo effect in many of the studies to date. But could the placebo effect really explain an increase in pregnancy rate from 16 percent to 33 percent? Positive thinking is powerful, but not that powerful.

History has shown that when concerns about the placebo effect are overestimated, patients can suffer. The controversy over folic acid serves as just one example: Initial research showing that folic acid could prevent birth defects was blighted by the same type of criticism, leading to many years of heated controversy.[31]

Thirty years after the initial discovery of folic acid's benefits, we know that the early doubts about the value of folic acid in preventing birth defects probably caused many tragic outcomes that could have been avoided if medical advice had kept pace with research.

If DHEA is as beneficial as the current research indicates, questioning the value of this supplement may deprive some women of the opportunity to conceive with their own eggs or may incur the financial, emotional, and financial burden of repeating entire IVF cycles countless times to conceive when the odds of success are very low. Women undergoing IVF deserve to have all the possible tools to increase their chance of success.

The IVF clinic that started the DHEA movement—CHR—has been routinely recommending DHEA for all patients with diminished ovarian reserve since 2007.[32] This means that women with low AMH or high FSH, or women over 40, are typically advised to take DHEA when preparing for IVF. The clinic monitors testosterone levels and starts the IVF cycle when DHEA has brought the testosterone level up to the optimal range. Many other IVF clinics also routinely recommend that DHEA should be offered to women with diminished ovarian reserve preparing for IVF.[33]

## Testing

To determine whether DHEA is likely to help in your particular case, it is useful to have your current level tested. The amount of DHEA itself in the bloodstream at any given time fluctuates widely, so doctors instead test for the sulfated version, DHEA-S, which reflects the storage form and changes less over time. It is also useful to test for testosterone at the same time, because if DHEA-S is in the mid-range but testosterone is low, your doctor may still advise supplementing with DHEA in order to support testosterone production.

The precise DHEA-S and testosterone level at which supplementation is justified is not entirely clear. In the absence of hard data guiding this decision, clinics typically like to see both levels at the higher end of the normal range for young women (although some prefer even higher levels for DHEA-S, such as 350 mcg/dL).

Normal DHEA-S Ranges for Women:

Age 18–29 years 44–332 mcg/dL (1.19–9.00 μmol/L)

Age 30–39 years 31–228 mcg/dL (0.84–6.78 μmol/L)

Age 40–49 years 18–244 mcg/dL (0.49–6.61 μmol/L)

Normal Testosterone Ranges for Women:

Testosterone (bioavailable): 0.8–10.0 ng/dL (0.03–0.35 nmol/L)

Testosterone (free): 0.3–1.9 ng/dL (0.01–0.07 nmol/L)

Testosterone (total): 8–60 ng/dL (0.3–2.1 nmol/L)

If your doctor recommends that you take DHEA, it is also helpful to regularly retest your DHEA-S and testosterone levels to ensure you are taking the correct dose to maintain optimum levels.

## Safety and Side Effects

Because DHEA is thought to increase testosterone, it may have side effects related to male hormones, including oily skin, acne, hair loss, and facial hair growth.[34] It can also result in longer cycles. Although some researchers have suggested that DHEA use may result in impaired insulin sensitivity, impaired glucose tolerance, liver problems, manic episodes, and other rare side effects,[35] these side effects have not been seen in the studies testing DHEA in the fertility context.

The CHR group has reported that in over a thousand patients supplemented with DHEA, they have not encountered a single complication of clinical significance.[36] The most commonly reported side effect among the patients at CHR taking DHEA was increased energy.[37] The randomized clinical study performed in Israel also found no significant side effects,[38] and additional studies outside the fertility context have reported that long-term use of DHEA is safe.[39]

DHEA can, however, interact with medications. For example, it can interact with diabetes medication and increase insulin sensitivity. DHEA is not appropriate for those with certain medical conditions, including bipolar disorder, or a history of hormone-sensitive cancer.

It is also worth noting that a high level of DHEA-S, which can occur after supplementing at the full dose for several months, can make laboratory tests for progesterone less accurate. The practical result of that is that progesterone levels may appear higher than they actually are.[40]

## DHEA and endometriosis

There has been very little research on the use of DHEA in women with endometriosis. As a result, it cannot be entirely ruled out that long-term use could theoretically worsen the condition by facilitating the production of various different hormones. Nevertheless, some IVF clinics are beginning to recommend the short-term use of DHEA to reverse the impact of endometriosis on ovarian reserve, apparently with good results.

In a recent case report, doctors describe a 24-year-old woman with endometriosis and diminished ovarian reserve, with a low AMH (0.64 ng/mL) and a low follicle count (three to four antral follicles). After three months of treatment with DHEA, folic acid, and vitamin D, her AMH increased to 1.2 ng/ml. She underwent another IVF cycle and 16 eggs were retrieved. Many of these eggs fertilized and she successfully conceived on the first embryo transfer.[41]

Another case report described similar results. This time, a

29-year-old woman with endometriosis had a history of four failed IVF cycles, with only a couple of eggs retrieved in each cycle. She had an AMH of 0.6 ng/mL and a follicle count of three to six. Her testosterone was also quite low. After six weeks of supplementing with CoQ10 and DHEA, her testosterone rose to the middle of the normal range and she began her fifth IVF cycle. This time the results were markedly different. Eight eggs were retrieved, of which six fertilized, resulting in five embryos. She conceived on the first embryo transfer and eventually gave birth to a healthy baby girl.[42]

## DHEA and PCOS

DHEA is generally not recommended for those with PCOS, since PCOS most often involves high testosterone levels. Yet in 2017, the Center for Human Reproduction reported a previously unknown subgroup of PCOS patients who may in fact benefit. These patients are characterized by the unusual combination of high AMH but low DHEA-S and low testosterone, likely due to adrenal autoimmunity. Dr. Gleicher has reported that DHEA was able to improve IVF outcomes in these patients.[43]

## Formulation and Dosing

In the United States, DHEA is readily available as a vitamin supplement. Ten years ago, a study found that the purity and potency of these supplements was quite inconsistent, with brands ranging from 0–150 percent of the labeled dose.[44] The situation appears to have improved, however. A more recent analysis of a variety of brands found that all contained approximately the amount listed on the label.

When choosing a brand, it is helpful (but not essential) to look for a brand that is labeled as containing "micronized" DHEA. This means the DHEA has been formulated in tiny microparticles to improve absorption.[45] Recommended brands include Fertinatal, Pure Encapsulations, and Douglas Laboratories.

The dose of DHEA most often recommended by fertility clinics and used in clinical studies is 25 mg, three times per day.[46] Because studies have so consistently used this dose, there is very little research about what dose is actually needed to have a beneficial effect, and it may in fact be less. That is why ongoing testing is helpful, to ensure you are taking the right amount to maintain optimal levels of DHEA-S and testosterone, and are not in fact taking more than you need. If you are undecided about whether you want to start taking DHEA, one option is to start with a lower dose, such as 25 mg once per day. For many women, this will be sufficient to bring testosterone levels into the optimal range within a few months.

The research on DHEA suggests that it may take several months for this supplement to have a beneficial effect. For many women, this raises the question of whether or not to start taking DHEA if an IVF cycle is scheduled for just a few weeks away. This is a difficult decision and one to discuss with your doctor, but a factor to keep in mind is that if you do start taking DHEA and your upcoming cycle fails, you may at least have a better chance of the next IVF cycle succeeding because by that time, you will have been taking DHEA for the recommended two or three months.

If you are trying to conceive through IVF, you can stop

taking DHEA either the day before egg retrieval or when you get a positive pregnancy test. Once you reach egg retrieval, the supplement has done its work and is no longer needed for that cycle, but some doctors advise patients to continue taking it until they get a positive pregnancy test, because multiple IVF cycles may be needed. If you are trying to conceive naturally or through IUI, DHEA is stopped once you get pregnant.

## Conclusion

DHEA is one of the most powerful tools we have to address age-related infertility and diminished ovarian reserve. Numerous randomized and placebo-controlled studies show that for those with diminished ovarian reserve, DHEA can dramatically increase the odds of getting pregnant. It likely boosts not only the number of eggs retrieved, but also the quality, thereby reducing the risk of miscarriage.

If you have been diagnosed with diminished ovarian reserve, have age-related infertility, an autoimmune condition, or a history of early miscarriage, it is helpful to get your DHEA-S and testosterone levels tested. If your levels are in the lower half of the normal range, talk to your doctor about taking a DHEA supplement to improve your chances.

# CHAPTER 10

# Supplements That May Do More Harm Than Good

*"If you trust Google more than your doctor then maybe it's time to switch doctors."*

— JADELR AND CRISTINA CORDOVA

O NE OF THE natural consequences of the medical community's failure to give women complete information on which supplements may improve egg quality is that women must turn to less reliable sources of information and often end up taking supplements that are not supported by any scientific evidence.

This book features a vast number of clinical and laboratory studies showing that certain supplements can improve fertility, but attention must also be given to the supplements many women are taking in the hope of improving egg quality that are either ineffective or unsafe, or that may actually worsen egg quality and fertility.

## Pycnogenol

Pycnogenol is a patented extract from pine bark that has been shown to have antioxidant properties. This antioxidant capacity has led some people to include pycnogenol on lists of supplements for egg quality, even though no evidence exists from any good-quality clinical trials. Because pycnogenol is a mixture of compounds not naturally found in the body, there is reason to be very cautious about its safety.

At the time of writing, there have not been any good-quality clinical studies showing that pycnogenol can improve egg quality or even that it is safe and lacks side effects. The company that makes pycnogenol, which has a website touting 40 years of research into this supplement, identifies countless studies on the use of pycnogenol for a variety of conditions, including male infertility, but not a single study on egg quality or female fertility.[1]

Given the lack of evidence, there is no reason to take pycnogenol when other, much better, antioxidant supplements are available to improve egg quality, such as CoQ10, vitamin E, and alpha-lipoic acid. These antioxidants are naturally found inside ovarian follicles, and their supplement forms have been widely studied for safety and side effects in many large, double-blind, placebo-controlled clinical trials.

## Royal Jelly

Royal jelly is a substance secreted by worker bees to provide food for the queen bee. This jelly is thought to contain hormones that make the queen bee extremely fertile and increase her lifespan. Based on this natural role, royal jelly has long been recommended as an alternative medicine in the fertility context. Just like pycnogenol, royal jelly is a mixture of compounds not naturally found in the human body.

At the time of writing, no good-quality clinical research supports the use of royal jelly in improving egg quality, and it has been found to occasionally cause life-threatening allergic reactions. These allergic reactions likely occur because royal jelly contains some of the same allergens found in bee venom.[2] In addition, because royal jelly contains a mixture of chemicals that act like hormones, it may have unpredictable effects and disrupt natural hormone balance.[3] Given the uncertain benefit and side effects, royal jelly cannot be recommended as part of a regime to naturally improve fertility.

## L-Arginine

L-arginine is another supplement that many women take in an effort to improve egg quality before IVF. Unlike pycnogenol and royal jelly, it is naturally found in the fluid of ovarian follicles, but that does not mean that taking extra in supplement form is necessarily beneficial for egg quality.

The theory behind using L-arginine to improve egg quality is that it increases the production of nitric oxide, which dilates blood vessels and therefore would be expected to increase blood flow to the ovaries and uterus, bringing with it hormones and nutrients that encourage follicles to grow.[4]

In one of the early studies aimed at improving IVF outcomes using L-arginine, the supplement did have the intended effect of improving blood flow.[5] L-arginine supplements were given to women who were considered "poor responders" in IVF. This condition is thought to be caused by declining egg numbers and quality, often due to age.[6]

Among the women taking L-arginine, fewer cycles were canceled, and an increased number of eggs were retrieved and embryos transferred. There were three pregnancies in the group taking L-arginine and no pregnancies in patients who did not take L-arginine; however, all three pregnancies resulted in early miscarriage—a clear sign that something may have been wrong with the quality of the eggs and embryos. Nevertheless, the authors concluded that L-arginine supplements might improve pregnancy rate in poor responders, who often have impaired blood flow.[7]

While this research seemed to bring good news, follow-up research by some of the same doctors a few years later revealed that L-arginine supplements may actually decrease egg and embryo quality. Unlike the first study, the follow-up study involved women with tubal infertility rather than poor responders. The researchers thought that L-arginine would offer the same benefits seen in poor responders by improving blood flow during IVF.

What they found was very unexpected. The women who received L-arginine instead of a placebo actually had fewer good-quality embryos and a lower chance of becoming pregnant.[8] The pregnancy rate per cycle was nearly halved (16.6 percent versus 31.6 percent), as was the pregnancy rate per embryo transfer (18.7 percent versus 37.5 percent). Embryo quality, measured based on the appearance of the embryo, was also negatively affected by L-arginine.

This research demonstrated that L-arginine supplements can significantly decrease egg and embryo quality. This decrease was thought to be caused by the very increase in permeability that was originally thought to make L-arginine beneficial. But instead of improving the conditions for follicle growth, this increase in permeability allowed hormones to get into the follicles too easily and too early in the egg development process, resulting in quick, intense, and inconsistent follicle growth.

One of the goals of IVF is to have a group of follicles mature steadily at the same time so that on the day of egg retrieval, they are all at the right stage of maturation and are ready to be fertilized. It may be that L-arginine causes some follicles to mature too quickly and chaotically.

Studies have also shown that nitric oxide, which is elevated after L-arginine supplementation, can decrease the level of cellular energy (ATP) and also increase the level of oxidizing molecules, both of which would be expected to damage eggs and embryos.[9] The doctors responsible for the study concluded that L-arginine supplements have a detrimental effect on embryo quality and the chance of becoming pregnant.

This result was probably not evident in their previous study with poor responders because the poor responders likely already had lower-than-normal nitric oxide levels, so L-arginine had the effect of bringing nitric oxide levels up to normal. Yet when this supplement was given to people with normal levels, L-arginine was very detrimental.

Even in the previous studies on poor responders showing an increase in egg numbers, the eggs may have all been very poor quality because each of the resulting pregnancies ended in early miscarriage.

More recent research by a separate group has confirmed the

link between L-arginine and poor egg and embryo quality. In this research, instead of giving women L-arginine supplements, researchers measured the level of L-arginine naturally found in the fluid of ovarian follicles in one hundred women undergoing IVF.[10]

The study revealed a strong link between excessive L-arginine levels in ovarian follicles and fewer eggs retrieved and fewer embryos. The women in this study had a variety of causes of infertility, including male factor infertility, damaged or blocked fallopian tubes, endometriosis, and unexplained infertility. The clear implication from this research is that a high level of L-arginine has a negative effect on the development of eggs and embryos. Another study also found that high nitric oxide levels are associated with implantation failure and fragmented embryos.[11]

With this research in mind, the only circumstance in which to consider taking L-arginine before egg retrieval is if you have been diagnosed as a poor responder and have had multiple failed IVF cycles due to an insufficient number of eggs maturing. Even then, there is very limited evidence that L-arginine can improve egg numbers and it may actually decrease egg quality. In anyone other than a poor responder, the evidence shows that L-arginine can reduce egg and embryo numbers and quality and is therefore not a recommended supplement before egg retrieval.

After egg retrieval, and while preparing for embryo transfer, taking L-arginine may actually have value. At that point we are no longer concerned about a potentially detrimental effect on the egg maturation process and we can take advantage of the ability of L-arginine to boost blood flow to the uterus, which may help develop a uterine lining that is more receptive to an embryo, as discussed in the next chapter.

## Conclusion

Many women are taking supplements such as pycnogenol, royal jelly, or L-arginine in the hope of improving egg quality or egg numbers. But there is little evidence of safety or efficacy, and these unproven supplements may actually exacerbate the problem of poor egg quality, particularly in the case of L-arginine.

# CHAPTER 11

# Preparing for Embryo Transfer

*"Waiting makes me restless. When I'm ready, I'm ready."*
— REBA MCENTIRE

I F YOU ARE trying to conceive through IVF, what else can you do after egg retrieval to improve the odds of your embryo implanting? This chapter explains which supplements may help improve your uterine lining, and the potential value of acupuncture in the lead-up to embryo transfer.

In recent years there has been a trend away from transferring fresh embryos in the same week as the egg retrieval, with many clinics instead preferring to freeze all embryos and wait a month to perform the first transfer. This approach is backed up by research finding that the uterine lining can be less receptive in the time after egg retrieval, with significantly lower implantation rates for fresh transfers compared to frozen.[1] (This is likely because of a negative impact of stimulation medications). By freezing all embryos, it is possible to perform a transfer when the endometrial lining is primed and ready for embryo implantation.

There have now been many studies confirming a higher chance of pregnancy and live birth for frozen embryo transfers.[2] As one example, this was seen in a 2017 study of almost three thousand IVF cycles at some of the top clinics in the United States (including RMA and Shady Grove).[3] The pregnancy rate for freeze-all cycles was 52 percent, compared to 45 percent for cycles with a fresh transfer. The advantage of performing frozen rather than fresh transfers was even more noticeable for women over the age of 35.

Of course, there may be unique circumstances that favor a fresh transfer in certain cases. If you have very few embryos and they do not appear to be developing well, your clinic may be concerned that they will not survive the freeze and may decide that a fresh transfer will give you the best chance.

If your clinic does advise freezing all embryos so you can take a break before the transfer, how can you use that time to best advantage? In the month before embryo transfer, which of the supplements discussed so far are worth continuing, and what else can you do to improve your uterine lining?

As a starting point, you should continue taking your prenatal supplement and vitamin D. Having adequate levels of these vitamins right from the start of pregnancy is important for the health of the baby. Vitamin D in particular is important for reducing the risk of miscarriage and preterm birth. If you have PCOS, your doctor may also advise you to continue taking myo-inositol, to reduce the risk of gestational diabetes.

Beyond those basic supplements, there are also a few other

supplements that may be specifically helpful in the preparation for embryo transfer, as this chapter explains.

## The Overarching Goal While Preparing for Transfer

Two of the most important factors that dictate whether an embryo will successfully implant are the quality of the embryo and the thickness of the uterine lining (known as the endometrium). By focusing on egg and sperm quality for several months, you will have already done everything possible to improve the quality of the embryo. It then becomes time to focus on improving the thickness of the uterine lining.

Numerous studies have found that when the lining is thinner than normal, the chance of an embryo implanting is much lower. In a 2016 study of frozen embryo transfers, the chance of a live birth rate for women with a lining of 9 mm or greater was over 32 percent, whereas for women with a lining of 8 mm or less, the chance of giving birth was just 24 percent.[4] A study published in 2018 found that the greatest negative impact occurs in women with a lining of less than 7mm.[5]

Having a thin lining is a particularly common problem in women trying to conceive through medicated IUI. That is because medications such as clomiphene citrate and letrozole can thin the lining, even more than the medications used in IVF. The consequence of this in the IUI context is still somewhat controversial though, with a recent study of women trying to conceive through medicated IUI finding no association between endometrial thickness and pregnancy rates.[6] Nevertheless, many studies in the IVF context have found that lining thickness does count, so it is likely worthwhile trying to do what we can to address this factor.

In addition, women with a thin lining appear to be more likely to have an ectopic pregnancy, with a study finding a 5 percent chance in women with a lining less than 8 mm, compared to just 2 percent in women with a lining over 15mm.[7] This provides all the more reason to consider supplements that may be able to support the development of a healthy uterine lining.

## Supplements for Lining Prep

Compared to the studies on egg quality, there has been comparatively little research on supplements to improve the uterine lining for embryo transfer. There is, however, some evidence that vitamin E and L-arginine are helpful.

In 2019, a randomized, placebo-controlled study of women with repeated implantation failure found that supplementing with vitamin E significantly improved lining thickness.[8] An earlier study, involving 60 patients with a thin lining, also found that supplementing with either vitamin E or L-arginine improved endometrial thickness in about half of patients.[9]

In that study, the doses used were 600 mg per day for vitamin E and 6 g per day for L-arginine. Although the women were assigned to receive either vitamin E or L-arginine to compare the effects, it may be even more effective to combine the two supplements, because they work in slightly different ways.

Vitamin E appears to be particularly useful because it boosts cell numbers in the uterine lining and promotes the development of new blood vessels. L-arginine likely works by dilating blood vessels and thereby improving blood flow.

Other than vitamin E and L-arginine, there is very little evidence for any further supplements. There is a possibility that CoQ10 can improve endometrial thickness, although this is far from certain. One study has reported an increase in endometrial thickness in women taking CoQ10,[10] but these women had PCOS and were being treated with clomiphene citrate, so it is not clear whether other women would see the same benefit.

CoQ10 could theoretically support lining development more generally by enhancing the function of mitochondria. It has been known since the 1960s that certain cells in the uterine lining suddenly develop so-called "giant mitochondria" at certain stages of the menstrual cycle. This suggests a greater need for energy production in the cells lining the uterus, which could be supported by providing additional CoQ10.

In addition, CoQ10 plays an important role in regenerating vitamin E back into its active form, so this may be one more way in which CoQ10 could further help lining preparation. Ultimately, however, there is little research confirming that CoQ10 is helpful when preparing for embryo transfer, so this supplement becomes a lower priority after egg retrieval.

## Further Measures for Lining Preparation

In addition to taking vitamin E and L-arginine (and possibly CoQ10), your doctor should be able to advise on further steps to support your lining. They will often prescribe additional estrogen, which has been proven effective in boosting lining thickness. Aspirin may also help make the uterine lining more receptive. For those with markedly thin lining, your doctor may prescribe Viagra suppositories, a relatively new treatment that is backed by several studies.[11] Viagra is thought to support lining development by boosting blood flow.

To improve your odds even further, your doctor may decide to perform a minor procedure known as a "scratch," in order to trigger some healthy inflammation, which is needed for implantation. Some doctors also suggest acupuncture to prepare for embryo transfer.

## The evidence for acupuncture

Acupuncture has long been used as a treatment for infertility, but researchers are still trying to determine whether it actually does improve IVF success rates. Many IVF clinics began recommending or offering acupuncture treatments in the early 2000s, following the publication of a high-profile study led by Dr. Wolfgang Paulus in Germany.[12] Dr. Paulus showed that women who received acupuncture 25 minutes before and after embryo transfer had a 43 percent success rate, compared to a 26 percent success rate for those who did not get acupuncture. Many other groups have since tried to replicate these findings, often with disappointing results.

Now almost twenty years later, when all the studies are pooled together, it appears there is little to no impact on the chance of pregnancy from just one or two acupuncture treatments around the time of embryo transfer.[13] Yet even just this isolated treatment may still have other benefits, with many physicians recommending acupuncture to IVF patients purely because it reduces stress and anxiety. It is not clear that stress actually impacts fertility as much as some may think, but relieving stress is a worthy goal in and of itself.

It is also clear that if stress relief is the goal, acupuncture works. Research has consistently found that in women undergoing IVF, acupuncture reduces the level of the stress hormone cortisol.[14] In 2009, Dr. Alice Domar, the Director of Mind/Body Services at Boston IVF and a well-known expert on natural approaches to improving fertility, also performed a study using the same acupuncture protocol as Dr. Paulus.[15] Patients were randomized to either lie quietly or receive an acupuncture treatment for 25 minutes before and after transfer. The study found no impact on pregnancy rates but concluded that "acupuncture patients reported significantly less anxiety posttransfer and reported feeling more optimistic about their cycle."

It is possible that this stress-relieving benefit may only be seen when acupuncture is available onsite at the IVF clinic. One study found that when women have to travel from the IVF clinic to a new location for their first acupuncture on the day of embryo transfer, the benefits seem to disappear.[16]

Rather than isolated acupuncture treatment on the day of embryo transfer, there may be much more value in receiving regular treatments several times per week during the IVF cycle itself and in the month before a frozen embryo transfer.

Although the evidence on that point is far from conclusive, there is some initial research suggesting that a series of acupuncture treatments may improve the odds in IVF cycles.[17] In one successful trial, patients received acupuncture twice per week for four weeks before egg retrieval, with additional treatments the day before and shortly after embryo transfer.[18] The pregnancy rate was significantly higher in the acupuncture group (53 percent) compared to controls (41 percent).

If indeed acupuncture can improve the odds of success in IVF, there are several possible explanations. One is that acupuncture may promote blood flow to the ovaries and uterus, encouraging follicle growth and the development of the uterine lining. It has also been suggested that acupuncture may improve fertility by triggering the release of beneficial endorphins and reducing stress hormones. Regardless of the precise way in which acupuncture brings benefits for those trying to conceive, it does appear that a series of regular treatments is needed, not just isolated sessions immediately before or after embryo transfer.

At the end of the day, acupuncture is one approach to try if your budget permits and if you find it relaxing. If, however, finding the time and money for acupuncture is going to be an added burden and one more source of stress, then it may not be right for you. There are a variety of other possible ways to reduce stress involved in the IVF process, such as yoga and meditation, with many good online resources: see www. itstartswiththeegg.com/resources.

CHAPTER 12

# Putting It All Together: Your Complete Supplement Plan

*"Forget past mistakes. Forget failures. Forget every-
thing except what you're going to do now and do it."*
WILLIAM DURANT

## Supplement Timing

**B**EFORE PROVIDING AN overview of possible supplement
plans for various fertility scenarios, there are some
generally applicable principles on the timing of when
to start and stop each supplement. (Always discuss supplement plans with your doctor first.)

### When to start

- If you are trying to conceive naturally, start the relevant supplements as soon as possible.

- If you are trying to conceive through IUI or IVF, you will benefit most if CoQ10, alpha-lipoic acid, N-acetylcysteine, vitamin E, and DHEA are started at least two to three months before your egg retrieval or insemination, if possible. For melatonin, the recent successful studies have started the supplement one month or two weeks before egg retrieval.

- If your IVF cycle is scheduled for less than two months away, there is likely still a benefit of starting supplements now. Some studies have found benefits from short-term supplementing, and if nothing else, the supplements can help you prepare for the next IVF cycle if your upcoming cycle is not successful.

- L-arginine can be started after egg retrieval, in preparation for embryo transfer.

- If you have a history of recurrent miscarriage, consider taking supplements for three months before trying to conceive again.

## When to stop

- Different IVF clinics recommend that patients stop CoQ10 either the day before egg retrieval, before embryo transfer, or once you get a positive pregnancy test. A reasonable middle-ground is to stop the day before embryo transfer. This may have the added advantage of promoting the development of the uterine lining. When taken during early pregnancy, CoQ10 may also help prevent miscarriages caused by antiphospholipid syndrome, although this is speculative at the moment and there is currently a lack of data on the safety of CoQ10 during pregnancy.

- Most other egg-quality supplements can be stopped the day before egg retrieval, because at that point they are no longer needed. This includes melatonin, alpha-lipoic acid, vitamin C, N-acetylcysteine, myo-inositol, and DHEA.

- If you have diminished ovarian reserve, your doctor may advise you to continue CoQ10 and DHEA until a positive pregnancy test, since multiple back-to-back IVF cycles may be needed.

- Vitamin E can be continued until embryo transfer, because it is helpful for preparing the uterine lining.

- Prenatals and vitamin D can be continued throughout pregnancy and until you stop nursing. It is wise to monitor your vitamin D levels occasionally during pregnancy to ensure you are taking the right dose.

- If you are trying to conceive naturally or through IUI, supplements are stopped when you get a positive pregnancy test (except your prenatal and vitamin D).

- If you have PCOS, your doctor may recommend that you continue taking myo-inositol during your pregnancy to prevent gestational diabetes.

For specific advice on other supplements to consider adding during pregnancy to support your baby's development, see www.itstartswiththeegg.com/sequel.

## Example Supplement Plans

Check with your doctor before beginning any new supplement
For recommended brands, please visit
**www.itstartswiththeegg.com/supplements**

## The Basic Plan

If you are just starting to think about getting pregnant and have no reason to expect any difficulty, you can likely shorten the time it takes to get pregnant and reduce the risk of miscarriage with the following approach:

- Start taking a daily prenatal multivitamin as soon as possible, ideally one that includes at least 800 mcg of methylfolate or natural food folate.

- Consider adding a daily CoQ10 supplement to enhance energy production inside developing eggs and possibly prevent chromosomal errors. The most effective form of CoQ10 is ubiquinol or Bio-Quinon, and the basic dose is 200 mg, preferably taken in the morning with food.

- Have your vitamin D level tested and consider supplementing with 4000–5000 IU of vitamin D3 per day if you are below the optimal target level (40 ng/ml or 100 nmol/L). If you have a significant deficiency, you can start with 10,000 IU per day for two weeks.

## Intermediate Plan: Difficulty Conceiving

If you are having trouble getting pregnant but have not yet moved on to treatments such as IUI or IVF, you can take a middle-ground approach and add some further basic supplements, with an emphasis on antioxidants. Studies have shown that women with unexplained infertility often have compromised antioxidant defenses in their ovarian follicles and that antioxidant supplements can reduce the time it takes them to conceive. If you decide to progress to IVF, you can then move to the advanced plan, discussed later in this chapter.

- Consider adding the following supplements:

  › A prenatal multivitamin containing at least 800 mcg of methylfolate or natural food folate

  › Ubiquinol: 400 mg per day—one 200 mg capsule with breakfast, one with lunch

  › Additional vitamin C (500 mg) and vitamin E (200 IU). You may also consider adding either alpha-lipoic acid or N-acetylcysteine for a stronger antioxidant boost.

- Ask your doctor to test you for vitamin D deficiency, celiac disease, and underactive thyroid. These three conditions often contribute to unexplained infertility and are typically overlooked by fertility specialists. They are also relatively easy to address.

- If your vitamin D is below the optimal target level (40 ng/ml or 100 nmol/L), consider supplementing with 4000–5000 IU of vitamin D3 per day. If you have a significant deficiency, you can start with 10,000 IU per day for two weeks.

## Intermediate Plan: Polycystic Ovary Syndrome or Irregular Ovulation

PCOS is one of the most common causes of infertility. Symptoms include weight gain, acne, facial hair, and irregular menstrual cycles or cycles longer than 35 days. PCOS causes infertility by disturbing normal ovulation and reducing egg quality. To improve egg quality and rebalance hormones:

- Consider taking the following supplements for two or three months before trying to conceive:

  › A prenatal containing 800 mcg of natural food folate or methylfolate

  › Myo-inositol: 4 g per day, divided into two doses—half in the morning and half at night

  › Ubiquinol: 400 mg per day—one 200 mg capsule with breakfast, one with lunch

  › R-alpha lipoic acid: 200 mg—preferably at least 30 minutes before a meal

  › N-acetylcysteine: 600 mg—any time

  › L-carnitine: 3 g per day—any time

  › Melatonin: 3 mg—bedtime (in women with

PCOS, melatonin appears to be useful even outside the context of IVF)

- Have your vitamin D level tested and consider
  supplementing with 4000–5000 IU of vitamin D3
  per day if you are below the optimal target level
  (40 ng/ml or 100 nmol/L). If you have a significant
  deficiency, you can start with 10,000 IU per day for
  two weeks.

### Advanced Plan: Endometriosis

Endometriosis impacts fertility in a variety of ways, but two
major components are inflammation and oxidative damage to
developing eggs. Research indicates it may be possible to counteract these problems to some extent with the right supplements.

- Consider taking the following supplements:
  › A prenatal with at least 800 mcg of natural food
    folate or methylfolate
  › CoQ10 (as ubiquinol or Bio-Quinon): 400 mg
    per day—one 200 mg capsule with breakfast, one
    with lunch. Some IVF clinics may recommend
    600 mg per day for difficult cases.
  › R-alpha lipoic acid: 300 mg—preferably at least
    30 minutes before a meal
  › N-acetylcysteine: 600 mg—any time
  › Vitamin C: 1000 mg—any time

> › If you are trying to conceive through IVF: mela-
> tonin, 3 mg at bedtime, starting two weeks to one
> month before egg retrieval.

- If you have had previous IVF cycles fail due to
a low number of eggs retrieved, or you have low
AMH or a low follicle count, have your DHEA-S
and testosterone levels tested. If your levels are not
in the higher end of the normal range for young
women, talk to your doctor about taking a DHEA
supplement for two or three months before your
next IVF cycle. There has been very little research
on the use of DHEA in women with endometriosis, but intial reports indicate that DHEA can help
address the negative impact of endometriosis on
ovarian reserve.

- Have your vitamin D level tested and consider supplementing with 4000–5000 IU of vitamin D3 per
day if you are below the optimal target level (40
ng/ml or 100 nmol/L). Some believe aiming for an
even higher target of 60 ng/ml may help reduce
the inflammation associated with endometriosis. If
you have a significant deficiency, you can start with
10,000 IU per day for two weeks.

### Advanced Plan: Recurrent Miscarriage

While there are various medical causes of recurrent miscarriage, including blood clotting and immune disorders, nearly
half of all early miscarriages are caused by chromosomal

errors in the egg. By improving your egg quality, you may be able to reduce the chance of chromosomal errors occurring and thereby reduce your risk of miscarriage.

- Consider taking the following supplements for two or three months before trying to conceive:
  › A prenatal with at least 800 mcg of methylfolate
  › CoQ10 (as ubiquinol or Bio-Quinon): 400 mg per day—one 200 mg capsule with breakfast, one with lunch
  › R-alpha lipoic acid: 200–300 mg—preferably at least 30 minutes before a meal
  › Vitamin E: 200 IU—any time
  › N-acetylcysteine: 600 mg—any time
  › If you have insulin resistance, myo-inositol: 4 g per day, divided into two doses—half in the morning and half at night
  › If you are trying to conceive through IVF, consider adding a melatonin supplement: 3 mg at bedtime, starting two weeks to one month before egg retrieval

- Ask your doctor to test you for underactive thyroid, a major cause of recurrent miscarriage. Studies have found that in women with autoimmune thyroid disease, treatment with an added thyroid hormone called levothyroxine reduces the miscarriage rate by more than 50 percent.

- Consider testing for celiac disease, particularly if you have any symptoms or a family history of celiac or autoimmune disease.

- Have your vitamin D level tested and consider supplementing with 4000–5000 IU of vitamin D3 per day if you are below the optimal target level (at least 40ng/ml or 100 nmol/L, although some believe a higher target is preferred to control inflammation). If you have a significant deficiency, you can start with 10,000 IU per day for two weeks.

- Consider having your DHEA-S and testosterone levels tested, particularly if age may be a factor or you have low AMH or a low follicle count. Supplementing with DHEA may help increase the number of eggs that mature properly each month and potentially prevent some of the chromosomal errors that cause miscarriage.

- Make sure your male partner is also taking a daily multivitamin containing methylfolate, a CoQ10 supplement (at least 200 mg of ubiquinol or Bio-Quinon), and the advanced sperm quality supplements discussed in chapter 14.

## Advanced Plan: Trying to Conceive Through IUI or IVF

If you have been diagnosed with diminished ovarian reserve or age-related infertility, or you need to pursue IVF or IUI for some other reason (such as endometriosis), you have the most to gain from an aggressive plan to improve egg quality.

- Consider taking the following supplements for two or three months before your next IVF cycle:
  - › A prenatal with at least 800 mcg of natural food folate or methylfolate
  - › CoQ10 (as ubiquinol or Bio-Quinon): 400 mg per day—one 200 mg capsule with breakfast, one with lunch. Some clinics may recommend 600 mg per day for difficult cases.
  - › R-alpha lipoic acid: 200–300 mg—preferably at least 30 minutes before a meal
  - › N-acetylcysteine: 600 mg—any time
  - › Vitamin E: 200 IU—any time. You may also decide to add vitamin C (500 mg) to boost antioxidant defenses even more.
  - › For IVF: melatonin, 3 mg at bedtime, starting two weeks to one month before egg retrieval
  - › As an optional extra, vitamin C: 500 mg—any time
- Have your DHEA-S and testosterone levels tested. If your levels are not in the higher end of the normal

range for young women, consider also taking a DHEA supplement for two or three months before your next IVF cycle. Look for a brand that is micronized such as Fertinatal, Pure Encapsulations, or Douglas Laboratories. The typical dose is 25 mg, three times per day, although you may require less.

- Ask your doctor to test you for underactive thyroid, a common cause of diminished ovarian reserve in younger women.

- Have your vitamin D level tested and consider supplementing with 4000–5000 IU of vitamin D3 per day if you are below the optimal target level (40 ng/ml or 100 nmol/L). If you have a significant deficiency, you can start with 10,000 IU per day for two weeks.

- Make sure your male partner is also taking a daily multivitamin containing methylfolate, a CoQ10 supplement (at least 200 mg of ubiquinol or Bio-Quinon), and the advanced sperm quality supplements discussed in chapter 14.

# Part 3

# THE BIGGER PICTURE

# CHAPTER 13

# The Egg Quality Diet

*"We are indeed much more than what we eat, but what we eat can nevertheless help us to be much more than what we are."*
— ADELLE DAVIS

TO MANY, IT will come as no surprise that diet can have a powerful influence on fertility. Numerous books have been written on the subject, but unfortunately this abundance of nutritional advice is typically based on general ideas of a "healthy diet" rather than solid scientific research. When we delve into the actual research on how diet impacts fertility, some surprising patterns emerge.

This chapter begins with the most powerful change you can make to your diet—a reduction in refined carbohydrates. This first step is critical to boosting egg quality and fertility.

## Carbohydrates and Fertility

One of the key goals of a fertility diet is to balance your blood sugar and insulin levels. We can do this by choosing the right kinds of carbohydrates and lowering overall carbohydrate intake, while increasing protein. To understand why this is so important, we need to briefly delve into what happens when we eat carbohydrates.

After consuming refined carbohydrates such as white bread, the starches are quickly broken down by enzymes in the digestive system. Because starch is nothing more than long chains of glucose molecules joined end to end, when starch is digested, the glucose is released into the bloodstream, triggering a rapid rise in blood glucose levels.

In refined carbohydrates, in which the grain has been broken apart and pulverized into tiny particles to make flour, the starch molecules are easily accessible to digestive enzymes, so they can be broken down very quickly.

By contrast, unrefined grains and seeds such as quinoa take much longer to break down because the starches are still wrapped up inside the grain or seed. As a result, the carbohydrates are digested more slowly, and the glucose molecules are released gradually over time. This means that the blood sugar response after eating whole, unrefined grains is much slower and steadier. Instead of a sudden spike in glucose levels, there is a slow climb.

One of the problems with a sudden spike in blood glucose levels is that it causes the pancreas to release a huge amount of insulin in an effort to get muscle cells to take up glucose from the bloodstream. This system is important because if all the extra glucose stayed in the bloodstream, it would quickly cause damage throughout the body. The glucose needs to be safely stored away inside muscles or converted into fat. Insulin directs this process by telling muscle and fat cells to soak up glucose.

The higher the blood glucose level, the more insulin is released. Over time, with repeated high levels of sugar and insulin, the cells become resistant to insulin's message to soak up glucose, a condition called "insulin resistance." Blood glucose levels remain high, the body compensates by making even more insulin, and chaos ensues.

All this sugar and insulin is a big problem for fertility because it disrupts the balance of other hormones that regulate the reproductive system.

One of the first studies showing this was published in 1999 by a group of researchers in Denmark.[1] In 165 couples trying to conceive, the researchers looked at a marker of average blood sugar levels over the preceding three to four months, called A1C. They found that women with high but still normal A1C levels were only *half* as likely to get pregnant over six months compared to women with lower A1C levels. This suggests that frequently having high blood sugar can compromise fertility.

This brings us to one of the most valuable sources of information on how nutrition affects fertility: the Nurses Health Study. This extraordinary study revealed several factors impacting fertility, the most powerful of which came from the type of carbohydrates in the diet. Before we discuss the specific findings of the Nurses Health Study, it is worth noting just how immense this study was.

The Nurses Health Study began in 1975 and followed thousands of nurses over several decades. It was originally designed to determine the long-term effects of birth control but quickly evolved into a much larger survey on the impact of lifestyle factors on health and disease, becoming one of the most comprehensive health studies ever performed.

In 1989, a second round of the Nurses Health Study was initiated in order to answer more detailed questions and explore specific health issues such as fertility—issues that could not be fully analyzed in the earlier part of the study. In this second round, more than 100,000 women participated. Every two years, these women answered detailed questions about their diet, exercise, and many other lifestyle factors, along with recording whether they got pregnant or had a miscarriage.

From this group of 100,000 women, scientists at the Harvard School of Public Health then selected a subgroup of more than 18,000 women who were trying to get pregnant and had not previously reported problems with infertility.[2] The researchers analyzed eight years of data from this subgroup to develop a picture of how nutrition could affect fertility. They did so by separating the women into two further subgroups: those who reported having ovulatory infertility (infertility caused by irregular ovulation or failure to ovulate) and those who did not. The researchers then compared the dietary patterns between both groups.

At the end of all this analysis, the Nurses Health Study revealed that while the total amount of carbohydrates in the diet was not connected to ovulatory infertility, the *type* of carbohydrates was very important. Women who ate more of the quickly digested carbohydrates that rapidly raise blood sugar were 78 percent more likely to have ovulatory infertility than women who ate slowly digested carbohydrates. Specifically, the particular carbohydrates linked to the highest risk of infertility were cold breakfast cereals, white rice, and potatoes; whereas brown rice and dark bread were linked to a lower risk of infertility.

For the purposes of the study, carbohydrates were categorized as "slow" or "fast" based on the glycemic index. This is
a measure of the rise in blood glucose levels over a specific
time period after eating a specific amount of carbohydrates. A
high-glycemic carbohydrate, which is typically highly refined,
is thus a "fast" carbohydrate that raises blood sugar levels too
much and too quickly. A low-glycemic carbohydrate, typically
minimally processed, is a "slow" carbohydrate.

The dramatic finding of the Nurses Health Study was that
women who followed a diet of low-glycemic/"slow" carbohydrates had a much lower rate of ovulatory infertility.

This is likely because high insulin levels impair ovulation
by disturbing the delicate balance of hormones in the ovaries.[3]
The net result is that even in normal, healthy women, elevated
insulin may contribute to problems with ovulation.

By modifying your diet to choose slow carbohydrates such
as unrefined grains over fast carbohydrates such as potatoes,
you may be able to balance blood sugar and insulin levels
and thereby rebalance the important hormones that regulate
ovulation.

Yet restoring ovulation is not the only reason to pay attention
to the amount and type of carbohydrates in your diet—high
insulin and blood glucose levels also compromise egg quality.

## Blood sugar, insulin, and egg quality

The negative effect of insulin on egg quality is particularly
apparent in the IVF context. This was seen when researchers
measured the levels of "advanced glycosylation end products,"
which are molecules that accumulate in the blood as a result

of high blood sugar levels over time.[4] They found that women with higher levels of these molecules had fewer eggs retrieved, fewer eggs fertilized, and fewer good-quality embryos. The pregnancy rate was also very different: 23 percent in women with normal blood sugar levels compared to just 3.4 percent in women with high levels.[5]

Importantly, this study was not testing women known to have a risk factor for insulin resistance but rather a variety of infertility causes, including tubal factor and unexplained infertility. This means that the results are likely relevant for all women trying to conceive, suggesting a general need to control blood sugar levels for optimal egg quality.

Delving further into the question of how exactly high blood sugar and insulin reduce egg quality brings us right back to the subject of earlier chapters: mitochondria. As explained in earlier chapters, mitochondria are the tiny power plants inside all our cells that produce energy in the form of ATP. ATP is critically important to egg development, and as a result, any disruption in mitochondrial function compromises the ability of eggs to mature and to process chromosomes properly.

Unfortunately, high blood sugar and insulin levels impair mitochondrial function.[6] This decreases ATP levels, which causes the cellular machinery that processes chromosomes to malfunction. We would therefore expect an increase in the rate of chromosomal abnormalities, and researchers have seen just that in animal studies. Eggs from diabetic mice are much more likely to have an incorrect number of chromosomes.[7]

All this information suggests that women with high blood sugar or high insulin levels who are undergoing IVF are at an increased risk of impaired embryo development and implantation failure. They may also have a higher risk of miscarriage.

## Insulin and miscarriage risk

Although often missed by doctors, there is a clear link between insulin resistance and the risk of miscarriage. More than a decade ago, scientists revealed that the rate of insulin resistance in women with recurrent pregnancy loss was nearly three times higher than normal.[8] Although the precise mechanism for this link is not well understood, research shows that high blood sugar or high insulin levels can significantly increase the risk of miscarriage.[9]

## Putting It All Together

The clear message of all this research is that out-of-control blood sugar and insulin levels are bad news for fertility—for *all* women trying to conceive. But there is good news too. Now that we understand the negative impact of high insulin levels, we have the opportunity to make a significant difference to fertility by getting our insulin under control.

The first step is to slightly reduce overall carbohydrate intake. This appears to have a powerful impact on IVF success rates, even in women without noticeable insulin or blood sugar problems. In one study, researchers asked twelve young, healthy women with previous failed IVF cycles to eat fewer carbohydrates and more protein.[10] On average, the women increased their protein intake from 15 percent of their calories to 27 percent. They also decreased their carbohydrate intake from 49 percent to 40 percent. The women followed this diet for two months before their next IVF cycle and the researchers then compared the outcomes to each woman's previous round of IVF.

The improvement was clear, particularly with respect to the percentage of eggs retrieved that made it to five-day embryo stage. While the women followed their normal diet, 19 percent of eggs developed into blastocysts, yet after two months of a lower carbohydrate and higher protein diet, 45 percent of eggs survived to the blastocyst stage. Ten out of the 12 women also became pregnant.

From this, the researchers concluded that "seemingly young healthy patients with poor embryo development can possibly increase the percentage of blastocyst formation by increasing their daily intake of protein and lowering their daily carbohydrate intake 2 months prior to their IVF cycle."

Importantly, this study indicates that the reduction in carbohydrates and increase in protein does not have to be extreme in order to improve egg and embryo quality. A good ratio appears to be around 40 percent of calories from carbohydrates, 30 percent from protein, and 30 percent from fat.[11] This represents a healthy, balanced diet, and many people will be able to easily reach these ratios by changing just one meal per day, such as having eggs for breakfast rather than toast or cereal.

To confirm that you are in the right ballpark, it may be helpful to use a macronutrient-tracking phone app for several days, such as Carb Manager. Alternatively, you can aim for approximately 50 grams of carbohydrates per meal, plus one snack of 20 to 30 grams of carbohydrates. (This will add up to 170–180 grams per day, which is 40 percent of calories for a woman eating 1800 calories per day.)

An even lower carbohydrate diet is likely helpful for those who are very overweight or have PCOS, diabetes, or insulin resistance. But for most women, it is probably not necessary or even beneficial to adopt a very low carbohydrate diet. In some cases, a ketogenic diet may even have negative consequences for fertility, by elevating cortisol levels and suppressing thyroid function.[12]

In the majority of cases, the goal is simply to maintain balanced blood sugar levels and to avoid the potentially harmful effects of very high blood sugar and insulin levels. Lowering overall carbohydrate intake is the first step to achieving this, but of course we should also remember that not all carbohydrates are created equal. By choosing the right kinds of carbohydrates, we can do even more to manage blood sugar and insulin levels, to help protect developing eggs.

## How to Choose Carbohydrates for Optimum Fertility

From a fertility standpoint, the best carbohydrates are those that are digested slowly and that only moderately raise blood sugar, preventing sudden bursts of insulin. This includes legumes, nuts, seeds, vegetables, and minimally processed whole grains such as quinoa, wild rice, brown rice, steel-cut oats, and buckwheat. Choosing more of these foods and minimizing foods made from highly processed or refined grains will help balance blood sugar and provide steady energy levels.

The next step is to reduce sugar, in all its forms. There is clear evidence that excess sugar consumption compromises fertility. As one example, a 2017 study by researchers at the Harvard

School of Public Health found that women undergoing IVF who typically drank sugared soda ended up with fewer eggs retrieved and fewer good-quality embryos.[13] Overall, the women who drank more than one glass of soda per day had a 16 percent lower chance of live birth per IVF cycle.

Even outside the IVF context, sugar compromises fertility. In 2018, researchers demonstrated that women who drank more than one sugar-sweetened beverage per day took longer to become pregnant.[14] Interestingly, the same was true for men, with soda consumption delaying the time to pregnancy of their partners.

Although it is clear that sugary drinks and candy should be avoided while trying to conceive, the question becomes how much further you need to go to avoid other sources of sugar, such as fruit.

The chemical differences between the types of sugars found in fruit, honey, table sugar, and high-fructose corn syrup are minimal—glucose, fructose, and sucrose all cause similar rises in blood sugar and insulin.[15] For that reason, it makes sense to minimize all types of sweeteners and foods with significant amounts of added sugar.

Whole fruit also contains some sugar, but it is likely fine to include in moderation. The sugar in fruit is packed together with fiber, which slows absorption and to some extent lessens the impact on blood sugar levels. Fruit also provides a range of beneficial antioxidants and vitamins with powerful fertility benefits.

In contrast, sugary drinks and added sweeteners have no redeeming nutritional qualities—they raise blood sugar and insulin levels without making you feel full and without providing any vitamins or other nutrients.

The best approach is therefore to avoid added sugars and to include small amounts of fruit. Most people will be able to include two servings of fruit per day. (With a serving referring to a small apple or banana, or a cup of berries). If you have PCOS and therefore need to control your blood sugar levels even more closely, it may be wise to limit fruit to just one serving per day and choose lower-sugar options such as berries.

If you find yourself needing a sweet treat and fruit simply will not do, a small amount of dark chocolate is a good choice. Also keep in mind that it is long-term daily habits that matter most. The occasional indulgence when you really need it is not worth feeling guilty about.

### What about High-Carbohydrate Vegetables?

Almost all vegetables are superfoods for fertility. The only ones to even pause over are starchy or sweet ones: potatoes, winter squash, pumpkin, sweet potatoes, carrots, yams, and corn. These vegetables will have a greater impact on blood sugar levels than other vegetables, but this impact is generally compensated for by the nutritional value they provide, so they can still be included in reasonable portions.

Potatoes and corn might be one exception, because they have a particularly noticeable impact on glucose levels, without providing a great deal of vitamins or antioxidants. By contrast, sweet potatoes, carrots, winter squash, and pumpkin are rich in beta-carotene, a vitamin A precursor that is very important to fertility. These brightly colored vegetables are also rich in many other vitamins and so are good nutritional choices.

## Other Benefits to Balancing Blood Sugar

A side benefit to cutting back on sugar and choosing slow carbohydrates over quick-release carbohydrates is that you will feel full longer and crave carbohydrates less. This is because the sudden bursts of insulin released to cope with high blood sugar levels will often drive blood glucose too low, leaving you craving another quick hit of carbohydrates.

With a steady rise in blood glucose levels, the relatively small insulin response will not drive blood glucose levels down so far, minimizing the peaks and valleys in your blood sugar levels. Your mood, energy level, and food cravings will likely improve, and if you are overweight, this strategy will probably also help you lose weight without feeling hungry. This can itself be a huge benefit for fertility—just a 5–10 percent weight loss in overweight women can often restore fertility.

## Is It Necessary to Eliminate Gluten or Dairy?

Gluten clearly contributes to infertility and miscarriage risk in those with celiac disease; that much is beyond doubt. The question is whether it is necessary for everyone else to avoid gluten and perhaps also dairy while trying to conceive.

There is some concern that both gluten and dairy can contribute to autoimmunity and inflammation in those with a sensitivity, even in the absence of celiac disease. As will be discussed further toward the end of this chapter, for those with endometriosis, a history of recurrent miscarriage driven by immune factors, or a pre-existing autoimmune disease, it probably does make sense to avoid gluten and dairy. For everyone else, these foods may not be problematic.

The typical advice to avoid dairy while trying to conceive is often based on a concern that the hormones present in milk could compromise fertility. Yet the studies so far have not found a clear link. We know from the Nurses Health Study that a higher intake of full-fat dairy was actually associated with a lower risk of ovulation disorder. In a more recent study of IVF outcomes, women with the highest dairy intake had the highest chance of live birth.[16]

You can of course choose to avoid gluten and dairy if you prefer a no-stone-unturned approach. There are numerous anecdotal reports of women battling infertility who were able to conceive after eliminating these foods. One option is to eliminate them for two weeks and see how you respond. If you feel better overall, that may indicate that you do indeed have a sensitivity and will benefit from avoiding gluten or dairy (or both) longer term.

### Boosting Fertility with a Mediterranean Diet

If the first principle of a fertility-friendly diet is balancing blood sugar, the second is adopting an overall Mediterranean-style diet. This diet, which is based on the traditional eating patterns in Greece, Spain, and Southern Italy, emphasizes fish, olive oil, legumes, and antioxidant-rich vegetables. It has long been hailed as one of the healthiest dietary patterns, shown to increase life expectancy and lower the risk of heart disease, cancer, and diabetes.[17]

Most importantly for our purposes, the Mediterranean diet also lowers inflammation.[18] This matters because there is a growing body of evidence tying inflammation to infertility and miscarriage, with a slew of new studies on this link published in 2018.[19] Before exploring the topic of inflammation, it is helpful to review what is perhaps the most persuasive reason to adopt a Mediterranean diet while trying to conceive: researchers have specifically found that eating this way can boost IVF success rates.

In 2018, researchers demonstrated that women who followed a Mediterranean-style diet for six months before IVF were much more likely to become pregnant.[20] The foods with the strongest links to improved success rates were vegetables, fruit, whole grains, legumes, fish, and olive oil.

This follows on from a previous important study on diet and IVF success rates, which surveyed 161 couples at an IVF clinic in the Netherlands. There, the researchers found that women who closely followed a Mediterranean diet before their IVF cycle had a 40 percent higher chance of becoming pregnant.[21] Again, the "Mediterranean diet" in the study was characterized by a high intake of vegetables, vegetable oil, fish, and legumes. The researchers suggested two ways in which these foods could improve pregnancy rates so dramatically. The first is a higher level of specific vitamins, such as folate, B6, and B12. The second is a higher level of certain fatty acids.

## Key vitamins in the Mediterranean diet

The theory that specific vitamins are partly responsible for the beneficial effect of the Mediterranean diet is supported by the fact that women who closely followed this way of eating in the Dutch IVF study had significantly higher levels of folate (found in grains and vegetables) and also somewhat higher levels of vitamin B6 and vitamin B12 (found in fish, dairy, eggs, and meat).

Each of these vitamins benefits fertility in a number of ways, but their biggest impact could be through reducing levels of a harmful amino acid called homocysteine. The more closely women followed the Mediterranean diet, the lower their homocysteine levels.

As described in earlier chapters, scientists have known for many years that a deficiency in folate or vitamin B12 causes the amino acid homocysteine to build up in the body, which in turn reduces the number and quality of eggs in IVF cycles and reduces embryo quality.[22] High homocysteine levels have also been linked to a high rate of miscarriage, by causing either chromosomal abnormalities or increasing the risk of blood clotting.[23]

The Mediterranean diet may therefore improve fertility by increasing levels of key fertility vitamins that detoxify homocysteine, thereby improving egg and embryo quality. A number of large-scale studies have now confirmed that a Mediterranean diet does indeed lower homocysteine levels.[24] This key benefit is likely to be particularly important for those with genetic variants in folate metabolism genes, such as MTHFR. These genetic variants are thought to contribute to the risk of infertility and miscarriage in large part by causing elevated homocysteine levels.

Vitamin B6 alone could also have a major impact on boosting fertility in women following a Mediterranean diet because research has found that supplementing with this vitamin can increase the chance of conception by 40 percent and decrease early miscarriage by 30 percent.[25] Vitamin B6 is found in particularly large amounts in fish, a key component of the Mediterranean diet.

## Fertility-friendly fats and oils

Another way in which a Mediterranean diet likely improves fertility and may even reduce miscarriage risk is by emphasizing anti-inflammatory fats and oils, particularly those found in fish, nuts, and olive oil.[26] In recent years, a wave of high-quality studies has demonstrated that these fats are beneficial for fertility, while saturated fats are likely harmful.[27]

In the IVF context, researchers have demonstrated that women with a sufficient level of omega-3 fats typically have higher-quality embryos.[28] They are also more likely to become pregnant. In 2017, Harvard researchers found that women with above-average levels of omega-3 fats in their blood had a much higher chance of conceiving through IVF.[29]

This study also made an important distinction about the type of omega-3 fats. The type found in plant sources (such as flaxseed oil) did not appear to have much impact. Only the specific omega-3s found in fish were linked to better odds of conceiving.

Even outside the context of IVF, studies have found that eating more fish appears to significantly improve fertility. And this applies to men too. As one example, a 2018 study tracked seafood consumption in five hundred couples that were trying to conceive naturally. The researchers found that 92 percent of couples that ate seafood more than twice a week were pregnant at the end of that year, compared to 79 percent among couples consuming less seafood.[30] Audrey Gaskins of the

Harvard School of Public Health commented that "our results stress the importance of not only female, but also male diet on time to pregnancy and suggests that both partners should be incorporating more seafood into their diets for the maximum fertility benefit."

An even larger study, this time involving two thousand women, also reported that women with sufficient omega-3 intake conceived sooner than those with a low intake.[31] The researchers noted this was likely because omega-3 fats reduce inflammation, support progesterone production, and increase uterine blood flow.

One interesting pattern to emerge in these recent studies is that above a certain level of omega-3 intake, consuming more does not confer any additional benefit. The threshold for improving fertility appears to be eating omega-3 rich fish approximately two times per week.

Most women who are trying to conceive eat much less. This is in part due to concerns over mercury, even though 90 percent of fish on the market is low in mercury. The commonly consumed fish that can have high mercury levels are swordfish and tuna. There are many other types of fish with very high omega-3 levels and negligible mercury, including salmon, sardines, and Atlantic mackerel.

Wild salmon is preferred over farmed, but farmed salmon from reputable sources is still a good choice. WholeFoods, for example, has strict standards to ensure the farmed salmon it sells is not contaminated with antibiotics or pesticides and does not harm the environment. The most cost-effective way to buy wild salmon is to purchase it frozen in bulk (such as from Costco) or in foil pouches.

If you do not eat seafood regularly, or only eat types of fish with much lower omega-3 levels, it may make sense to add a low-dose fish oil supplement. This can be considered an insurance policy, but the studies to date have not proven that supplements will achieve the same benefits as eating fish, at least in women. In men, fish oil supplements have been shown to improve sperm quality. A reasonable dose is approximately 700–1000 milligrams per day of omega-3s. Nordic Naturals is one of the highest-quality brands.

To further optimize fertility, the best type of oil to use is olive oil. This is a key component of the overall Mediterranean diet pattern and likely a major reason why this diet boosts IVF success rates.[32] Olive oil is not only rich in antioxidants such as vitamin E but also contains a type of monounsaturated fat known as oleic acid. Oleic acid is one of the main fats found naturally in developing eggs, and it appears to play an important role in egg development.[33]

A 2017 study found that women with higher levels of oleic acid in their bloodstream had more mature eggs retrieved before IVF.[34] Other fats found in olive oil, such as linoleic acid, have also been linked to improved fertility.[35] Nuts, seeds, and other plant-based oils are also rich in linoleic acid.

In contrast, saturated fats, which are typically found in coconut oil, butter, and red meat, appear to negatively effect egg development.[36] A high intake of red meat has been associated with lower embryo quality.[37] In contrast, a diet high in fish and olive oil but low in red meat was found to support early embryo growth.[38]

Taken as a whole, the research indicates that we can significantly improve fertility by aiming for a higher intake of fish, olive oil, nuts, and seeds, and a somewhat lower intake of saturated fat and red meat.

Research published in 2018 indicates that rebalancing fat intake in this way may be particularly important for those with variants in folate metabolism genes, such as MTHFR. Specifically, the study found that a higher consumption of fish and a higher ratio of monounsaturated to saturated fat results in lower homocysteine levels.[39] As discussed above, one way these genetic variants may contribute to infertility and miscarriage is by increasing homocysteine levels. This research suggests that a Mediterranean diet may therefore be able to reduce the impact of MTHFR variants on fertility.

## The Mediterranean diet and miscarriage

An anti-inflammatory Mediterranean diet is also likely to be particularly helpful for preventing the miscarriages that are not caused by chromosomal errors in eggs. Most of the strategies discussed in previous chapters have focused on preventing chromosome-related miscarriage, but there are also steps you can take to address other potential causes.

Some women show a pattern of repeated pregnancy losses even where testing shows no chromosomal abnormality in the fetus. Clearly there is something else going on in these cases. Recent studies show that one likely culprit is inflammation.

In a 2018 study, researchers in Spain tested a dozen different blood markers in a group of women who were under 30 and had each experienced at least three miscarriages. The women with a history of recurrent miscarriage showed two clear differences compared to the controls: a higher level of inflammation (shown by a marker called C-reactive protein) and lower vitamin D levels.[40]

Vitamin D calms inflammation and is obviously important for preventing miscarriage, as discussed in chapter 4. But we can also lower inflammation through diet. Numerous studies have found that following a Mediterranean diet can lower inflammation, and specifically lower C-reactive protein.[41] Shifting toward this type of diet is therefore likely to be helpful in reducing the risk of miscarriage driven by inflammation.

The term "inflammation" generally refers to nonspecific immune activity, where the immune system rages with no particular target. But in some cases, recurrent miscarriage can also be caused by more direct immune activity, such as particular antibodies directed against the body's own proteins. This type of immune activity is referred to as "autoimmunity" and in the miscarriage context includes antiphospholipid antibody syndrome.

If you have lost one or more pregnancies and test positive for these or other antibodies, you may ultimately need immune-suppressing medication (and/or anti-clotting medication) to reduce your risk of miscarriage, but there are also additional dietary strategies to consider, as the next section explains.

## A Modified Fertility Diet for Autoimmunity, Endometriosis, and Immune-Mediated Miscarriage

If you fall into the group of women with fertility problems involving the immune system, you may benefit by modifying your diet even further. This group includes those with:

- A preexisting autoimmune condition (such as thyroid disease, psoriasis, lupus, multiple sclerosis, Crohn's disease, or ulcerative colitis)

- Endometriosis

- Miscarriage with immune factors (such as antiphospholipid antibody syndrome)

In all of these conditions, the immune system is reacting inappropriately to the body's own molecules and often triggering a very high level of inflammation. This inflammation can compromise egg quality and potentially contribute to miscarriage risk.

It is therefore worthwhile to pay particular attention to dietary factors that influence general inflammation, as discussed above. This means an even greater focus on reducing sugar and saturated fats while emphasizing anti-inflammatory vegetables and healthy fats from fish and olive oil. But many women with immune system disruptions will benefit from going even further, by eliminating foods that are typically regarded as healthy but can sometimes trigger immune reactions in those with a sensitivity. Here, the two main culprits are gluten and dairy.

Gluten and dairy are now widely recognized as worsening autoimmune disease in those with a sensitivity. As a result, even the most conservative endocrinologists now often recommend that women with autoimmune thyroid conditions go gluten and dairy-free while trying to conceive. Studies have also found that a gluten-free diet reduces pain in 75 percent of patients with endometriosis.[42]

For women with miscarriages driven by immune factors, a gluten-free diet may also be helpful. We know that celiac disease is a common cause of recurrent miscarriage, but it is possible for gluten to contribute to inflammation and immune disruption even if you only have a nonceliac sensitivity. (There are lab tests that can detect such sensitivities.)

Dr. Jeffrey Braverman, a renowned reproductive immunologist who specializes in treating recurrent miscarriage, notes that is important to take gluten sensitivity very seriously in the treatment of recurrent pregnancy loss. Although not all women with recurrent pregnancy loss will be sensitive to gluten, Dr. Braverman comments that "Overall you can never go wrong with being off gluten."

Dairy is another food that can potentially be problematic, simply because it is one of the most common food allergens. Eliminating both gluten and dairy can therefore go a long way toward calming the immune system in those with immune-driven fertility issues.

For those with more severe autoimmune diseases, there are of course further steps you can take if you choose. Diet can have a profound effect on autoimmune disease, as I have now witnessed firsthand by resolving my own debilitating psoriatic arthritis after a 15-year battle. (In my case, this condition caused extreme joint instability in my spine and hips, which is why I used a gestational surrogate. It was not until several years later that I finally learned how to control my autoimmune condition through diet—as explained in my 2017 book *The Keystone Approach: Healing Arthritis and Psoriasis by Restoring the Microbiome.*)

One typical recommended diet for those with autoimmune disease is the autoimmune paleo (AIP) diet, which emphasizes animal proteins, fruits, vegetables, coconut oil, and animal fats, while excluding grains, legumes, and common allergens such as nuts, eggs, and dairy.

Some components of this diet, such as avoiding allergens, are likely to be helpful for many with autoimmune disease, but there are certain aspects of the AIP diet that are counterproductive.

The latest scientific research shows that adding more red meat, coconut oil, and ghee, as many people do while following the AIP diet, can actually significantly increase inflammation. By contrast, a Mediterranean-based diet is much better at calming the immune system.

When we piece together all the various bodies of research on diet and autoimmunity, it appears that the best approach is to start with a Mediterranean-based diet and modify it by eliminating some of the foods that can be problematic for those with autoimmunity, such as grains, soy, corn, nuts, eggs, and dairy.

> For allergen-free, low-carbohydrate Mediterranean diet recipes, see **www.itstartswiththeegg.com/recipes**.

## Alcohol and Fertility

The question of whether alcohol compromises fertility has been plaguing researchers for decades. In 1998, a small but highly publicized study reported that consuming just one to five alcoholic drinks per week could significantly reduce the odds of conceiving.[43] Yet this study involved just four hundred women. Much larger studies have now been done and the results have been more reassuring.

A study of 40,000 women found reduced fertility only with more than 14 alcohol drinks per week.[44] The same result was evident in a 2016 study of six thousand women, with researchers concluding that "consumption of less than 14 servings of alcohol per week seemed to have no discernible effect on fertility."[45]

It should be noted that these studies were performed in the context of women trying to conceive naturally, so the results do not necessarily extend to women with pre-existing fertility problems who are trying to conceive through IVF.

In the context of IVF, moderate alcohol consumption may be slightly more problematic, but the effect still appears to be relatively small. In 2011, researchers at Harvard Medical School surveyed more than two thousand couples undergoing IVF. They found that compared to women reporting fewer than four alcoholic drinks per week, women drinking more than this amount had a 16 percent lower chance of a live birth.[46] Similar results were reported in 2014 by researchers in Spain.[47]

More recently, in one of the largest studies to date, researchers followed more than 12,000 women in Denmark who were trying to conceive through IVF. The study reported only a small drop in the chance of a live birth for women who were heavy drinkers (more than seven drinks per week), with a 20 percent chance of live birth per cycle compared to 22 percent for nondrinkers.[48] (Almost exactly the same trend was evident for male drinking.)

Another Harvard study, published in 2017, found that up to

12 grams of alcohol per day made no difference to the chance of live birth after IVF.[49] A small glass of wine contains 14 grams of alcohol, so the threshold level in this study would be equivalent to six drinks per week.

Of course, it is still safer to err on the side of caution and keep alcohol intake to an absolute minimum, but the research as a whole indicates that the occasional glass of wine is not going to significantly reduce your odds of getting pregnant.

The latest research also indicates that occasional alcohol consumption before pregnancy does not increase the risk of miscarriage or stillbirth. Here we have to make a careful distinction. Numerous studies have indicated that drinking regularly *during* pregnancy can increase the risk of miscarriage, likely because alcohol interferes with fetal development.[50] However, low to moderate alcohol consumption *before* you become pregnant is not as troubling.

That was the finding of a 2016 report from the Nurses Health Study, based on more than 27,000 pregnancies. The researchers concluded that *pre*pregnancy alcohol intake was not related to risk of miscarriage or stillbirth.[51] This study was limited to women without a history of pregnancy loss, however other researchers have commented that there is no greater link between alcohol intake and recurrent miscarriage.[52]

The most cautious approach is obviously to abstain from alcohol while trying to conceive. That is still the recommendation of the Centers for Disease Control, which states that "there is no known safe amount of alcohol use during pregnancy or while trying to get pregnant." But it appears the CDC's primary concern with alcohol consumption while trying to conceive is that a woman may be pregnant without knowing it, since most pregnancies are not discovered for four to six weeks. Consuming alcohol during that interval is problematic for a variety of reasons, but what if you have just had a failed IVF cycle or a pregnancy loss, or know for a fact that you are not currently pregnant? The most recent evidence suggests that a glass of wine at that point might be a reasonable choice.

## Caffeine and Fertility

Another controversial issue is the amount of caffeine that is safe while trying to conceive. Here again, the major concern is whether caffeine increases miscarriage risk.

It has been known for many years that consuming several cups of coffee per day *during* pregnancy can significantly increase the risk of miscarriage. Unfortunately, the same appears to be true for the time before pregnancy.

A 2018 study from more than 15,000 pregnancies found that compared to women with no prepregnancy coffee intake, those who drank four or more cups per day before pregnancy had a 20 percent higher chance of miscarriage.[53]

The risk was not as pronounced for the women drinking fewer coffees each day, but even a lower intake still raised the risk of miscarriage. That finding is consistent with prior studies, which reported that the miscarriage risk begins to rise even at 50 to 150 milligrams of caffeine per day during pregnancy.[54] Translating that into real-world terms, the amount of caffeine in a single cup of coffee is typically around 100 to 200 mg. (A Starbucks Tall brewed coffee has 260 mg of caffeine, while a double-shot cappuccino has 150 mg.) Many people also underestimate the amount of caffeine in tea. A cup of green tea typically contains around 25 mg of caffeine, while black tea often contains around 50 mg per cup. The studies therefore indicate that miscarriage risk begins to rise with just one cup of tea or less than half a cup of coffee per day.

In addition, even though most studies have found no impact on fertility, some research does suggest that caffeine can make it more difficult to get pregnant. A Yale study revealed that women who used to drink tea or coffee in the past but stopped prior to fertility treatment had a higher pregnancy and live birth rate than current tea and coffee drinkers.[55] Another study also found a correlation between caffeine and a decrease in the number of good-quality embryos during IVF.[56]

So while it is probably not absolutely necessary to stop drinking tea and coffee altogether, there is reason to be quite cautious about how much caffeine you are consuming. One cup of tea or half a cup of coffee each day may not have a huge impact, but gradually switching to decaffeinated tea and coffee is an even safer choice. (Stepping down gradually over a few weeks will prevent withdrawal headaches.) When making decaf coffee at home, it might also be preferable to buy organic beans that have been decaffeinated by the "Swiss Water Process" rather than chemical solvents. For recommended brands, see www.itstartswiththeegg.com/coffee.

## The Overall Fertility Diet

Clear scientific evidence has established that certain types of carbohydrates harm fertility by causing spikes in blood sugar levels, which in turn cause major hormonal disruptions and reduce egg quality. Reducing overall carbohydrate intake and choosing more whole, natural foods such as quinoa, wild rice, and legumes, will help keep blood sugar levels steady. This in turn can balance a range of hormones and significantly improve egg quality.

Recent research has also revealed that the general pattern of the Mediterranean diet is associated with improved fertility, with significantly higher success rates in IVF. There is very good reason for this: the Mediterranean diet emphasizes vegetables, healthy fats, legumes, and seafood, all of which are higher in specific vitamins and fatty acids associated with lower inflammation and improved fertility.

## Action Steps

To boost your fertility, choose a diet based on

- slowly digested carbohydrates from unprocessed foods such as quinoa, wild rice, steel-cut oats, buckwheat, lentils, and other legumes;

- limited amounts of starchy, brightly colored vegetables such as sweet potato, winter squash, pumpkin, and carrots;

- leafy greens and other nonstarchy vegetables;

- moderate amounts of fruit (two servings per day);

- lean, unprocessed protein such as fish, chicken, and beans; and

- healthy fats such as olive oil, avocado, nuts, and seeds.

You can further improve your egg quality and fertility by avoiding

- refined carbohydrates such as white bread and highly processed breakfast cereals;

- added sugar and other sweeteners;

- gluten and dairy if you have an inflammatory or autoimmune condition (including recurrent miscarriage, endometriosis, or thyroid disease); and

- caffeine and alcohol (although you can probably allow yourself an occasional glass of wine when you know you are not pregnant).

# CHAPTER 14

# The Other Half of the Equation: Sperm Quality

*"The difference between the impossible and the possible lies in a man's determination."*
—TOMMY LASORDA

FOR ANY COUPLE trying to conceive, sperm quality matters. It matters even more when the female partner has poor egg quality or very few eggs to retrieve in an IVF cycle, whether due to age-related infertility or some other cause. In these situations, a woman simply cannot afford to waste one of her few good eggs on suboptimal sperm. It falls to the male partner to make sure his contribution to the equation is as good as possible. New research is also revealing that sperm quality may be a major contributor to recurrent miscarriage, providing all the more reason for men to do everything possible to support their sperm quality in the months before conception.

Fortunately, there are several ways to improve sperm quality—using supplements and other strategies that are backed up by years of scientific research. But first, we need to dispel some of the pervasive myths surrounding male fertility.

## Myth No. 1:
## Difficulty conceiving can usually be
## attributed to the female partner

Contrary to popular belief, male infertility contributes to nearly 50 percent of all cases in which a couple has difficulty conceiving.[1] The misconception that female infertility is more common may be due to the fact that treatment in a fertility clinic typically entails many procedures, medications, and injections for women but not for men.

Even though the female partner is nearly always the main focus of fertility treatments such as IUI and IVF, in many cases these treatments are needed only to circumvent problems with sperm quality. Yet even with these advanced fertility treatments as a work-around, low sperm quality can remain a limiting factor and can increase the risk of miscarriage.

In the end, whether a couple is trying to conceive naturally or through IVF, the male side of the equation is critically important and rarely given the attention it deserves.

Part of the problem is that traditional semen analysis done in fertility clinics is woefully inadequate. A conventional semen analysis will look at three standard measures (together termed "semen parameters"):

1. Sperm Count/Concentration: the number of sperm per unit of volume of semen

2. Motility: the sperm's ability to swim properly toward the egg

3. Morphology: the percent of sperm that have a normal shape and overall appearance

While a problem in any one of these parameters will definitely make it more difficult to conceive, this traditional semen analysis does not tell the whole story. The screening may come back perfectly normal, even though poor sperm quality remains a barrier to conceiving. This is because the traditional measures do not adequately investigate the extent of damage to the DNA inside the sperm.

The latest research suggests that DNA quality matters more than conventional semen parameters. The term "DNA quality" reflects whether the DNA has individual mutations, extra or missing copies of chromosomes, or physical breaks in the DNA strands. This last type of damage results in fragmentation of the chromosomes and is the type of damage that can actually be measured now using advanced sperm quality analysis (discussed further below).

Each type of damage to DNA causes its own set of problems: decreased chance of fertilization, decreased chance of the embryo successfully implanting to become a pregnancy, and increased risk of the child being born with a serious birth defect or a genetic disease caused by a new spontaneous mutation.

Evidence is emerging that DNA damage in sperm also increases the risk of miscarriage. In one recent study, researchers found much higher levels of DNA damage in sperm from couples with a history of unexplained miscarriage, suggesting that this DNA damage could be a contributing factor to pregnancy loss.[2] In 2019, a study reported that in couples with a history of recurrent miscarriage, the average level of DNA damage in sperm was two-fold higher.[3] A 2017 study also found that the degree of DNA damage in sperm has a major impact on the chance of conceiving through IVF.[4]

In short, the extent of DNA damage in sperm is an important factor for any couple trying to conceive, but it is especially critical to address in couples with a history of miscarriage or failed IVF cycles. In these cases, it can also be helpful to pursue testing for DNA fragmentation. One of the most accurate tests for this is known as the Sperm Chromatin Structure Assay (SCSA), available through SCSA diagnostics. The cost is approximately $500 but may be covered by insurance and could potentially prevent the cost of a failed IVF cycle.

## Myth No. 2:
## Male fertility does not decline until after age 50

The reality is that a typical 45-year-old man is significantly less fertile than a man 10 years younger, with sperm quality beginning to decline as early as age 35.[5] A large part of the reason for this decline is that sperm from older men have more DNA breakage, DNA mutations, and other chromosomal abnormalities.[6] In fact, DNA fragmentation in sperm doubles from ages 30–45.[7]

The age-related decline in male fertility is often overlooked.

Many people wrongly assume that while an older mother is more likely to miscarry or have a baby with a birth defect such as Down's syndrome, the father's age has no impact on these outcomes. Research shows that fathers over the age of 40 have a 20 percent greater chance of having a baby with a serious birth defect.[8] Higher levels of DNA damage in sperm also more than double the risk of miscarriage.[9]

It is not just the DNA inside sperm that suffers with increasing age. Sperm motility starts to decline at age 35, and age also negatively impacts sperm count and morphology.[10]

But it's not all bad news. Research also shows that some of this decline can be prevented and reversed, with several studies finding that older men following a healthy diet and taking the right supplements have sperm quality similar to younger men. This brings us to the most significant myth of all.

## Myth No. 3:
## Nothing can be done to improve sperm quality

Decades of scientific research contradict this widely held belief and show that it is possible to improve sperm quality and even improve the quality of the DNA within the sperm. Doing so has a whole host of benefits: increasing the chance of conceiving (whether naturally or in conjunction with assisted reproduction such as IVF) and reducing the risk of miscarriage and birth defects.

To understand what you can do to improve sperm quality, it helps to first understand how sperm become damaged in the first place.

The cycle of producing each sperm takes a little over two

months.[11] During this time, many different environmental and lifestyle factors can impact the process, for better or worse. Yet by far the most important factor impacting sperm quality during this time is oxidation.

Oxidation is a chemical reaction in the body that is analogous to metal rusting or an apple turning brown. As sperm are produced, a normal, healthy level of oxidation takes place as a result of biological processes, while an army of defenders stops this oxidation from getting out of control. The defense system includes antioxidants such as vitamins C and E (semen contains a particularly high concentration of vitamin C), along with special enzymes that exist solely to protect sperm against oxidative damage.

When lifestyle factors such as toxin exposure or vitamin deficiencies cause too much oxidation or compromise the antioxidant defense system, the result is oxidative damage, which is thought to be a contributing factor in up to 80 percent of all cases of male infertility.[12]

Oxidation impacts the conventional semen parameters (sperm count, motility, and morphology) as well as the amount of damage to sperm DNA.[13] Research at the Cleveland Clinic has confirmed that men with high levels of oxidation in semen have more extensive DNA fragmentation and fewer normally functioning sperm.[14]

Medical problems such as infections, blockages, and enlarged veins (varicocele) account for about a quarter of cases of male infertility.[15] If you are affected by one of these conditions, you may need medication or a minor surgical procedure to improve your sperm quality. Yet such conventional medical treatment does not obviate the need to also pay attention to lifestyle and nutritional factors that can improve sperm quality.

The reality is that natural approaches to improving sperm quality may be even more critical in men with urological conditions, because many conditions contribute to infertility by causing an increase in oxidative damage to sperm.[16]

Improving sperm quality may also be particularly critical when the female partner has poor egg quality. Unlike sperm, eggs have specialized machinery that can repair DNA damage, which allows eggs to overcome some of the negative effect of damaged sperm. Yet the DNA repair process only works effectively in good-quality eggs. An egg from an older woman may not be able to adequately repair the DNA damage from poor-quality sperm, making it even more difficult to conceive.[17]

The good news is that for most men, sperm quality is at least partly within your control through vitamin supplements and other simple steps you can take to guard against oxidative damage and thereby protect your fertility.

## How to Improve Your Sperm Quality

### Take a Daily Antioxidant Supplement

The single most important thing you can do to improve sperm quality is to take a daily supplement containing a combination of vitamins and antioxidants. Dozens of studies have clearly established that taking a daily antioxidant supplement improves sperm quality and increases the chance of conceiving.[18] This is true for couples trying to conceive naturally and those undergoing fertility treatment.

One systematic review of the research in this area, analyzing

34 prior studies, determined that men who take antioxidant supplements had more than a four times higher chance of their partner conceiving. There was also nearly a five times higher chance of a live birth when compared to men not taking anti-oxidants.[19] And no studies reported evidence of harmful side effects from the antioxidant therapy used.[20]

Some research suggests that antioxidants may be particularly powerful when infertility is caused by DNA damage within sperm. In one study, men with elevated DNA fragmentation were given vitamins C and E daily for two months following a failed attempt to achieve fertilization by ICSI (an approach similar to IVF, but sperm are injected directly into the eggs).[21] The researchers found an extraordinary improvement in the next attempt, with the clinical pregnancy rate jumping from 7 percent to 48 percent.

Different studies use different combinations of antioxidants, but the ones that have been studied the most in this context are vitamin C, vitamin E, zinc, folate, and selenium.[22] Vitamins C and E act directly as antioxidants, while zinc, folate, and selenium prevent oxidation in more complex ways, such as by assisting antioxidant enzymes. A deficiency in zinc or folate can also directly cause increased DNA damage.[23]

While many studies have tried to find out which of these vitamins (or which combination) help the most, you can cover all bases and probably get the most benefit by simply taking a daily multivitamin. A multivitamin designed specifically for men is a good option because it will probably contain more selenium.

If there is a history of recurrent miscarriage or failed IVF cycles, it is important to take a multivitamin that contains methylfolate, rather than synthetic folic acid. That is because new research has found a possible link between recurrent miscarriage and genetic defects in folate metabolism genes in the father.[24] Such defects likely contribute to miscarriage risk by impacting DNA quality in sperm.[25]

> For recommended multivitamin brands, see
> **www.itstartswiththeegg.com/male-supplements**.

Ideally, you will start taking a multivitamin two or three months before trying to conceive, but boosting your antioxidant levels for any time period before trying to conceive is likely to be beneficial.

## Add a Coenzyme Q10 Supplement

Although a multivitamin is the best starting point, there are additional antioxidants you can add for greater protection of sperm quality. The most useful is probably CoQ10—a vital antioxidant molecule found in just about every cell in the body. It is particularly beneficial for sperm quality because it is not just an antioxidant but also a critical component of energy production.

Researchers have known for many years that there is a link between sperm quality and the level of CoQ10 naturally present in semen. Men with lower CoQ10 levels tend to have a lower sperm count and poor motility.[26]

In recent years, several different randomized, double-blind, placebo-controlled studies have determined that taking a

CoQ10 supplement improves sperm concentration, motility, and morphology.[27] A recent study also found that the combination of CoQ10, antioxidants, and vitamin B12 not only improved traditional semen parameters but also significantly improved the integrity of DNA in sperm.[28]

One way in which CoQ10 is thought to improve sperm quality is by increasing the activity of antioxidant enzymes.[29] It also enhances cellular energy production. Sufficient energy in the form of a molecule called ATP is absolutely critical for sperm production and motility. Cells can only make ATP when they have enough CoQ10. Although not yet proven, it is therefore likely that CoQ10 supplements improve sperm quality by optimizing energy production. What has been proven is that CoQ10 can prevent oxidative damage to DNA in sperm,[30] providing reason enough to add this supplement.

When choosing a brand of CoQ10, a good form to take is known as ubiquinol (as explained in chapter 6), and the usual recommended dose is 200 mg per day.[31] For couples with particularly severe fertility issues, a dose of 400 mg may be more effective.

### Advanced Sperm Quality Supplements

In cases where sperm quality is known to be an issue, or there is a history of failed IVF cycles or recurrent miscarriage, it is likely helpful to go further and add several additional supplements that have been found to improve sperm quality. The most effective supplements are

- Alpha-lipoic acid

- Omega-3 fats (in fish oil)

- L-carnitine

Each of these supplements is backed up by clear scientific evidence. As just one example, a randomized, double-blind, placebo-controlled study found that when men took alpha-lipoic acid each day for 12 weeks, there was a significant improvement in the total sperm count, sperm concentration, and motility levels.[32]

The recommended dose is 600 milligrams per day for a standard alpha-lipoic acid supplement. If you choose a supplement that is in the form of R-alpha lipoic acid, it is likely sufficient to take 200 to 300 milligrams per day.

Double-blind, placebo-controlled trials have also found that omega-3 fish oil supplements improve sperm quality, with a particular improvement in DNA damage.[33] In a 2016 study, when men took a fish oil supplement for three months, the average percentage of sperm with DNA damage decreased from 22 percent to 9 percent.[34] The dose used in this study was 1500 mg of fish oil, containing 990 mg of DHA and 135 mg of EPA per day. For a similar dose, take two capsules of Nordic Naturals DHA Xtra.

Where testing shows that sperm motility is a concern, another useful supplement is L-carnitine. Randomized studies have found that on average, L-carnitine can improve motility by 8 percent and morphology by 5 percent.[35] Yet in men with a significant degree of oxidative damage to sperm, carnitine has a much greater impact. In those cases, it can increase the total number of motile sperm by more than two-fold.[36] As a result, carnitine appears to be especially effective in men with poor sperm quality caused by varicocele.[37] The recommended dose is 1000 mg per day.

There is an alternative form of carnitine available in supplement form, called acetyl-l-carnitine. The body naturally maintains an equilibrium between the two forms and studies have found that taking either can improve sperm quality.[38] L-carnitine may be preferred simply because it has been studied more extensively.

Although taking all of these supplements for several months is no doubt inconvenient, it can make a dramatic difference to the chance of success. It is often well worth the sacrifice in order to save your partner from the physical and emotional toll of yet another failed IVF cycle or pregnancy loss.

## Boost Your Antioxidant Levels Through Diet

To take full advantage of the power of antioxidants to boost sperm quality, it is a good idea to also maximize the antioxidants in your diet. The value in doing so is borne out by years of scientific research finding that men with a diet higher in antioxidants are more likely to produce sperm with the correct number of chromosomes and tend to have improved semen parameters such as sperm count and motility.[39]

As just one example, a recent study found that men with higher fruit and cereal intake had better sperm quality.[40] One of the nutrients likely to be responsible for this benefit is folate, which is found in particularly large amounts in fruit, vegetables, and fortified cereal.

While all women trying to conceive are told to take folate

supplements, researchers now understand that folate is imperative for men too. It plays a critical role in protecting sperm DNA.[41]

A recent study in California revealed that other antioxidants found in food may even prevent or reverse the increase in sperm DNA damage associated with aging. The study, which involved men having no known fertility problems, found that men with the highest total intake of vitamin C, vitamin E, zinc, and folate (from food and supplements) had much less sperm DNA damage.[42]

In fact, the men with the highest intake of these had sperm DNA quality similar to the younger men. This extraordinary finding suggests that we may be able to prevent a large part of the decline in fertility and increased risk of miscarriage and birth defects as men age.

A nutritious diet is important because it is likely that the specific antioxidants found in multivitamins are just a small percentage of the vast array of antioxidants found naturally in food. One additional antioxidant shown to be helpful for sperm quality but unlikely to be present in your typical multivitamin is lycopene.[43] This powerful antioxidant is found in tomatoes and becomes particularly concentrated once tomatoes are cooked, such as in tomato paste.

Other powerful antioxidants include anthocyanins, which give berries their dark purple color, and beta-carotene, found in sweet potatoes and carrots. Additional well-known sources of antioxidants are green tea and dark chocolate, although little is known about how these antioxidants relate to sperm quality. Until we know more about which antioxidants are most beneficial, the best approach is to eat a wide variety of fruits and vegetables, with a particular focus on the most brightly colored varieties, which are typically higher in antioxidants.

It is also particularly useful to choose fruits and vegetables that are naturally lower in pesticide residues. This includes papaya, pineapple, mango, honeydew melon, avocado, cabbage, onion, peas, and broccoli. In a recent study by researchers at the Harvard School of Public Health, men who ate more of these low-pesticide fruits and vegetables had a 169 percent higher total sperm count and a 173 percent higher sperm concentration.[44]

Beyond antioxidants, a persuasive body of research also indicates that the dietary factors discussed in detail in chapter 13 apply to men too. In particular, the studies show that reducing sugar and red meat intake, while eating more fish and unrefined whole grains, can have powerful benefits for male fertility.[45]

## Cut Back on Alcohol

There is no doubt that heavy alcohol intake is associated with poor sperm quality,[46] but the evidence is much less consistent when it comes to the impact of moderate alcohol consumption. While many studies have shown no effect, some studies have reported a link between even moderate alcohol consumption by men and reduced fertility, particularly in the IVF context.

One study by researchers at the University of California evaluated whether male alcohol use during the in vitro fertilization program affected the reproductive outcome. The researchers found that the risk of not achieving a live birth more than doubled for men who drank one additional drink per day.[47] In this study, the effect on live birth rate appeared to be due in large part to an increased miscarriage rate for couples in which men drank alcohol in the month before the IVF cycle.

A more recent study in men attending a fertility clinic in Brazil found that alcohol consumption decreased sperm count, sperm motility, and fertilization rate.[48] Alcohol intake is known to increase oxidative stress throughout the body,[49] providing one explanation for how alcohol may negatively impact sperm.

While the occasional single glass of wine may have little effect, beyond this amount it may be worth exercising caution, particularly if you face an uphill battle trying to conceive.

## Reduce Your Exposure to Environmental Toxins

The power of lifestyle factors to influence sperm quality does not end with diet. Everyday environmental toxins are thought to be a major contributing factor to the oxidative stress that is seen in up to 80 percent of infertile men. Toxins often cause increased oxidation by compromising the activity of antioxidant enzymes, along with a host of other harmful effects on sperm quality.

Over 80,000 chemicals are registered for use in the United States, yet only a small percentage have ever been analyzed for safety and even fewer for reproductive harm. Within the soup of chemicals we are all exposed to on a daily basis, it is not yet clear which toxins cause the most problems for men trying to conceive. However, so far, the toxins with the clearest evidence of harm to sperm quality are the same ones shown to harm

developing eggs: phthalates and BPA. They are both ubiqui-
tous chemicals that have long been known to disrupt hormone
activity (so called "endocrine disruptors").

## Phthalates

Phthalates are a group of chemicals called "plasticizers" that
are used in everything from cologne to laundry detergent to
air freshener to soft, flexible plastic made from vinyl or PVC.
As explained in more detail in chapter 3, these chemicals are
banned in children's toys, and some phthalates are banned in
personal care products in Europe, but overall very little has
been done to curb the quantity of phthalates we are exposed
to on a daily basis. This is despite the fact that scientists
have known for more than 20 years that these chemicals are
absorbed into the body and interfere with critical hormones.

By acting as endocrine disruptors, phthalates cause a range
of harmful effects, including genital malformations in baby
boys exposed in utero. After many years of heated controversy, it now appears to be well established that phthalates also .
damage sperm in adult men.[50]

The concentration of phthalates that men are commonly
exposed to has been shown to cause DNA damage in sperm
while also reducing sperm quality by traditional measures.
The damage may occur in a variety of ways, including altering
hormone levels and causing oxidative stress. Specifically,
higher phthalate levels have been linked to lower levels of testosterone and other hormones involved in male fertility.[51] A
large study involving more than 10,000 people also revealed
a link between higher levels of phthalates and more extensive
oxidative stress throughout the body.[52]

Ultimately, even a small decline in sperm quality caused by phthalates may translate into a significant reduction in fertility. At the 2013 meeting of the American Society of Reproductive Medicine, researchers presented the results of a study investigating the relationship between phthalate levels and odds of conceiving in five hundred couples. The researchers found that men who had the highest levels of phthalates in their bodies were 20 percent less likely to impregnate their partners over the course of a year.[53]

Men can reduce their exposure to phthalates by minimizing the use of vinyl/PVC in the home; switching to shampoo, shaving cream, and deodorant labeled as "phthalate-free" (such as those made by Every Man Jack, Burt's Bees, and Caswell-Massey); and avoiding unnecessary fragrance such as cologne and fragranced laundry detergent. Minimizing processed food and eating more food that is prepared at home from natural ingredients can also help dramatically reduce phthalate exposure.

## BPA

Bisphenol A, or BPA for short, is another toxin that poses a potential danger to male fertility. This chemical, and its closely related cousins, are commonly found in canned food, reusable plastic food storage containers, and the coating on paper receipts. Researchers have long been suspicious of BPA because it is an endocrine disruptor known to mimic the effects of estrogen.

In one of the earliest studies on the question of BPA and sperm quality, researchers at the University of Michigan found that higher urinary BPA levels were linked to lower sperm count, motility, and morphology, and a greater percentage of sperm DNA damage.[54]

Other studies have since confirmed that men with higher levels of BPA are more likely to have low sperm count and poor sperm quality.[55] In addition, animal studies have directly observed that exposure to BPA at levels equivalent to the amount humans are exposed to on a daily basis interferes with sperm production and causes DNA breakage in sperm.[56]

Even though some controversy still remains over the impact of BPA on sperm quality, there is now more than enough evidence to warrant caution. The most important practical steps are to avoid canned and highly processed foods and replace plastic kitchenware with glass or stainless steel, as discussed in more detail in chapter 2.

## Lead and other heavy metals

There is no question that lead poses a danger to human health. Fortunately, government action has significantly reduced lead in our environment. Even so, a little extra care is warranted if you are trying to conceive, because researchers have found that men with higher lead levels tend to have a significantly lower sperm count and a greater percentage of abnormal sperm.[57]

A good way to reduce your exposure is to use a water filter certified to remove lead. For advice on specific brands, see the Environmental Working Group's online water filter buying guide.[58] Old paint is another source of possible lead exposure, so consider buying a test kit if your home has older, crumbling paint. Removing your shoes at the door is another good step to take because research has found that dirt tracked in from outside is the major source of lead in house dust.

To manage some of the risk from various other chemicals in the environment that could also contribute to poor sperm quality, you can err on the side of caution by minimizing the use of home pesticides, garden weed killer, and insect sprays. You should also exercise caution if you have a hobby or profession that involves welding or the use of pesticides or organic solvents such as form-aldehyde. If you are particularly concerned about environmental toxins, the Environmental Working Group website has advice on how to avoid a dozen common endocrine disruptors, including fire retardants and arsenic (summarized at the end of chapter 3).[59]

## Chemicals in commercial lubricants

Research has recently revealed yet another group of chemi-cals that can interfere with fertility: those found in lubricants. Studies show that most lubricant brands significantly decrease sperm motility and increase DNA fragmentation.[60] It is there-fore important to choose a brand that is specifically designed for couples trying to conceive. In a 2014 study that compared 11 different lubricants, the brand with the least negative impact on sperm function was Pre-Seed.[61]

## Keep Your Distance from Cell Phones

Although commonly dismissed as a myth, scientific research actually does show that keeping a cell phone in your pocket could negatively impact sperm quality. Researchers at the Cleveland Clinic found that the use of cell phones decreases sperm count, motility, viability, and morphology, with a greater impact caused by a longer duration of daily exposure.[62] The same researchers also found that when sperm samples were exposed to radiation from a cell phone for one hour, there was a significant decrease in sperm motility and viability, and an increase in signs of oxidation.[63]

The radiofrequency electromagnetic waves emitted by cell phones are thought to damage sperm through a combination of heat generated by the electromagnetic waves and other effects, likely including oxidative stress.[64] These effects all depend on the cell phone being in very close physical proximity, so you can decrease your exposure by keeping your cell phone out of your pocket whenever possible.

## Stay Cool

Researchers have known for more than 40 years that elevated temperatures impair sperm quality. The impact of heat on sperm quality is readily apparent from the effect of a fever, which causes a drop in sperm count and motility.[65] The longer the fever, the worse the impact on sperm quality.

Other factors also increase temperature where it matters: sitting all day, taking hot baths or showers, and wearing tight-fitting underwear.[66] In one six-month study, researchers witnessed a 50 percent decrease in sperm parameters in men wearing tight-fitting underwear. Sperm parameters improved after subjects switched to loose-fitting underwear.[67]

Many fertility clinics advise men to avoid hot baths and showers in the week before sperm sample collection, but we know there are other ways to avoid overheating, such as taking regular breaks from sitting and wearing loose-fitting underwear. We also know that a week could be too short. The full process of sperm production takes over two months, and it is likely that early stages of sperm production are just as vulnerable to heat. The longer you can keep things cool, the better.

## Action Plan for Sperm Quality

- Take a daily multivitamin, ideally starting several months before trying to conceive. For couples with a history of failed IVF cycles or miscarriage, it is best to choose a brand that contains methylfolate rather than synthetic folic acid.

- To reduce DNA damage in sperm and improve sperm count, motility, and morphology, consider adding the following supplements:

  › CoQ10 (as ubiquinol or Bio-Quinon): 200 mg per day with breakfast. For couple with serious difficulties, consider increasing to 400 mg per day.

  › Fish oil: two capsules of Nordic Naturals DHA Xtra or equivalent to provide at least 900 mg of DHA

  › R-alpha lipoic acid: 200–300 mg per day, preferably on an empty stomach, but can be taken with breakfast if more convenient

  › L-carnitine: 1000 mg, with or without food

- Further boost your vitamin and antioxidant levels with a diet rich in brightly colored fruits and vegetables.

- Limit sugar and red meat intake, while eating more fish and unrefined whole grains.

- Reduce alcohol consumption, particularly in the lead-up to IVF.

- Take steps to reduce your exposure to toxins known to damage sperm: phthalates, BPA, lead, and the chemicals in commercial lubricants.

- Keep your cell phone out of your pocket when you can.

- Stay cool where it counts.

# Author's Note

**E**GG QUALITY HAS such profound implications for fertility that all women who are trying to conceive deserve to know what they can do to protect their own egg quality. If you found this book useful please help spread the word to other women who are struggling with infertility.

My hope is that the information provided in this book will allow others to overcome fertility challenges caused by poor egg quality and finally realize their dream of having a healthy baby. In short, I hope that others can be as fortunate as I have been. My own success story is pictured on the back cover of this book: my beautiful baby boy at ten days old.

For more success stories, research updates, and answers to common questions, please join my monthly email newsletter group: www.itstartswiththeegg.com/email-updates

# References

Scientific Publications are available from the National Institutes of Health database at www.ncbi.nlm.nih/pubmed

## Introduction

1 Wright VC, Chang J, Jeng G, Macaluso M. Assisted reproductive technology surveillance—United States, 2003. MMWR Surveill Summ. 2006 May 26;55(4):1-22.

2 Stagnaro-Green A.Thyroid antibodies and miscarriage: where are we at a generation later? J Thyroid Res. 2011;2011:841949.

3 Thangaratinam S, Tan A, Knox E, Kilby MD, Franklyn J, Coomarasamy A. Association between thyroid autoantibodies and miscarriage and preterm birth: meta-analysis of evidence. BMJ. 2011 May 9;342:d2616.

4 Sugiura-Ogasawara M, Ozaki Y, Katano K, Suzumori N, Kitaori T, Mizutani E. Abnormal embryonic karyotype is the most frequent cause of recurrent miscarriage. Hum Reprod. 2012 Aug;27(8):2297-303 ("Sugiura-Ogasawara 2012").

5 Macklon NS, Geraedts JP, Fauser BC. Conception to ongoing pregnancy: the 'black box' of early pregnancy loss. Hum Reprod Update. 2002 Jul-Aug;8(4):333-43 ("Macklon 2002").

## Chapter 1: Understanding Egg Quality

1 Sugiura-Ogasawara M, Ozaki Y, Katano K, Suzumori N, Kitaori T, Mizutani E. Abnormal embryonic karyotype is the most frequent cause of recurrent miscarriage. Hum Reprod. 2012 Aug;27(8):2297-303; Macklon NS, Geraedts JP, Fauser BC. Conception to ongoing pregnancy: the 'black box' of early pregnancy loss. Hum Reprod Update. 2002 Jul-Aug;8(4):333-43

2 Macklon 2002.

3 Hassold T, Hall H, Hunt P. The origin of human aneuploidy: where we have been, where we are going. Hum Mol Genet. 2007;16(Spec No. 2):R203–R208. ("Hassold and Hunt 2007"); Macklon 2002; Sher G, Keskintepe L, Keskintepe M, Ginsburg M, Maassarani G, Yakut T, Baltaci V, Kotze D, Unsal E.Oocyte karyotyping by comparative genomic hybridization provides a highly reliable

method for selecting "competent" embryos, markedly improving in vitro fertilization outcome: a multiphase study. Fertil Steril. 2007 May;87(5):1033-40.

4   Fragouli E, Alfarawati S, Goodall NN, Sánchez-García JF, Colls P, Wells D. The cytogenetics of polar bodies: insights into female meiosis and the diagnosis of aneuploidy. Mol Hum Reprod. 2011 May;17(5):286-95. ("Fragouli 2011").

5   van den Berg MM, van Maarle MC, van Wely M, Goddijn M. Genetics of early miscarriage. Biochim Biophys Acta. 2012 Dec;1822(12):1951-9; ("van den Berg 2012").
Macklon 2002

6   Macklon 2002.

7   Suguira-Ogasawara 2012.

8   Kushnir VA, Frattarelli JL. Aneuploidy in abortuses following IVF and ICSI. J Assist Reprod Genet. 2009 Mar;26(2-3):93-7; Kim JW, Lee WS, Yoon TK, Seok HH, Cho JH, Kim YS, Lyu SW, Shim SH. Chromosomal abnormalities in spontaneous abortion after assisted reproductive treatment. BMC Med Genet. 2010 Nov 3;11:153; van den Berg 2012

9   Macklon 2002.

10  Allen EG, Freeman SB, Druschel C, Hobbs CA, O'Leary LA, Romitti PA, Royle MH, Torfs CP, Sherman SL. Maternal age and risk for trisomy 21 assessed by the origin of chromosome nondisjunction: a report from the Atlanta and National Down Syndrome Projects. Hum Genet. 2009 Feb;125(1):41-52.

11  Fragouli 2011; Macklon 2002.

12  Pellestor F, Andréo B, Anahory T, Hamamah S. The occurrence of aneuploidy in human: lessons from the cytogenetic studies of human oocytes. Eur J Med Genet. 2006 Mar-Apr;49(2):103-16; Fragouli 2011; Macklon 2002.

13  Kuliev A, Zlatopolsky Z, Kirillova I, Spivakova J, Cieslak Janzen J. Meiosis errors in over 20,000 oocytes studied in the practice of preimplantation aneuploidy testing. Reprod Biomed Online. 2011 Jan;22(1):2-8.

14  Fragouli 2011.

15  Fragouli 2011.

16  http://www.colocrm.com/AboutCCRM/SuccessRates/2011statistics.aspx

17  Schoolcraft WB, Fragouli E, Stevens J, Munne S, Katz-Jaffe MG, Wells D. Clinical application of comprehensive chromosomal screening at the blastocyst stage. Fertil Steril. 2010 Oct;94(5):1700-6.

18 Katz-Jaffe MG, Surrey ES, Minjarez DA, Gustofson RL, Stevens JM, Schoolcraft WB. Association of abnormal ovarian reserve parameters with a higher incidence of aneuploid blastocysts. Obstet Gynecol. 2013 Jan;121(1):71-7.

19 Yang Z, Liu J, Collins GS, Salem SA, Liu X, Lyle SS, Peck AC, Sills ES, Salem RD. Selection of single blastocysts for fresh transfer via standard morphology assessment alone and with array CGH for good prognosis IVF patients: results from a randomized pilot study. Mol Cytogenet. 2012 May 2;5(1):24.

20 Munné S, Held KR, Magli CM, Ata B, Wells D, Fragouli E, Baukloh V, Fischer R, Gianaroli L. Intra-age, intercenter, and intercycle differences in chromosome abnormalities in oocytes. Fertil Steril. 2012 Apr;97(4):935-42.

21 Hassold T, Hunt P. Maternal age and chromosomally abnormal pregnancies: what we know and what we wish we knew. Curr Opin Pediatr. 2009 Dec;21(6):703-8.

22 Nagaoka SI, Hassold TJ, Hunt PA. Human aneuploidy: mechanisms and new insights into an age-old problem. Nat Rev Genet. 2012 Jun 18;13(7):493-504; Fragouli 2011;

23 Bentov Y, Yavorska T, Esfandiari N, Jurisicova A, Casper RF. The contribution of mitochondrial function to reproductive aging. J Assist Reprod Genet. 2011 Sep;28(9):773-83.

24 Van Blerkom J. Mitochondrial function in the human oocyte and embryo and their role in developmental competence. Mitochondrion. 2011 Sep;11(5):797-813. ("Van Blerkom 2011").

25 Van Blerkom 2011.

26 Shigenaga MK, Hagen TM, Ames BN. Oxidative damage and mitochondrial decay in aging. Proc Natl Acad Sci USA. 1994 91:10771-8.

27 Eichenlaub-Ritter U, Wieczorek M, Lüke S, Seidel T. Age related changes in mitochondrial function and new approaches to study redox regulation in mammalian oocytes in response to age or maturation conditions. Mitochondrion. 2011 Sep;11(5):783-96; Van Blerkom 2011.

28 Interview with Dr. Robert Casper, published in The Spectator, 11/19/2011. http://www.spectator.co.uk/features/7396723/resetting-the-clock/

## Chapter 2: How BPA Impacts Fertility

1 Dr. Patricia Hunt, personal communication. 2/6/2014.

2 Hunt PA, Koehler KE, Susiarjo M, Hodges CA, Ilagan A, Voigt RC, Thomas S, Thomas BF, Hassold TJ. Bisphenol a exposure causes

meiotic aneuploidy in the female mouse. Curr Biol. 2003 Apr
1;13(7):546-53. ("Hunt 2003").

3   Dr. Patricia Hunt, personal communication. 2/6/2014.

4   Hunt 2003.

5   vom Saal FS, Akingbemi BT, Belcher SM, Birnbaum LS, Crain
DA, Eriksen M, Farabollini F, Guillette LJ Jr, Hauser R, Heindel JJ,
Ho SM, Hunt PA, Iguchi T, Jobling S, Kanno J, Keri RA, Knudsen
KE, Laufer H, LeBlanc GA, Marcus M, McLachlan JA, Myers
JP, Nadal A, Newbold RR, Olea N, Prins GS, Richter CA, Rubin
BS, Sonnenschein C, Soto AM, Talsness CE, Vandenbergh JG,
Vandenberg LN, Walser-Kuntz DR, Watson CS, Welshons WV,
Wetherill Y, Zoeller RT. Chapel Hill bisphenol A expert panel
consensus statement: integration of mechanisms, effects in animals
and potential to impact human health at current levels of exposure.
Reprod Toxicol. 2007 Aug-Sep;24(2):131-8. ("vom Saal 2007").

6   Lang IA, Galloway TS, Scarlett A, Henley WE, Depledge M,
Wallace RB, Melzer D. Association of urinary bisphenol A
concentration with medical disorders and laboratory abnormalities
in adults. JAMA. 2008 Sep 17;300(11):1303-10; Shankar A, Teppala
S. Relationship between urinary bisphenol A levels and diabetes
mellitus. J Clin Endocrinol Metab. 2011 Dec; 96(12):3822-6; Silver
MK, O'Neill MS, Sowers MR, Park SK. Urinary bisphenol A and
type-2 diabetes in U.S. adults: data from NHANES 2003-2008.
PLoS One. 2011;6(10):e26868.

7   Melzer D, Rice NE, Lewis C, Henley WE, Galloway TS.
Association of urinary bisphenol a concentration with heart
disease: evidence from NHANES 2003/06. PLoS One. 2010 Jan
13;5(1):e8673.

8   Calafat AM, Ye X, Wong LY, Reidy JA, Needham LL. Exposure
of the U.S. population to bisphenol A and 4-tertiary-octylphenol:
2003-2004. Environ Health Perspect. 2008 Jan;116(1):39-44.

9   Stahlhut RW, Welshons WV, Swan SH. Bisphenol A data in
NHANES suggest longer than expected half-life, substantial
nonfood exposure, or both. Environ Health Perspect. 2009
May;117(5):784-9.
Vandenberg LN, Chahoud I, Heindel JJ, Padmanabhan V,
Paumgartten FJ, Schoenfelder G. Urinary, circulating, and tissue
biomonitoring studies indicate widespread exposure to bisphenol
A. Environ Health Perspect. 2010 Aug;118(8):1055-70.

10  Kitamura S, Suzuki T, Sanoh S, Kohta R, Jinno N, Sugihara K,
Yoshihara S, Fujimoto N, Watanabe H, Ohta S. Comparative study

of the endocrine-disrupting activity of bisphenol A and 19 related compounds. Toxicol Sci. 2005 Apr;84(2):249-59; Welshons WV, Nagel SC, vom Saal FS. Large effects from small exposures. III. Endocrine mechanisms mediating effects of bisphenol A at levels of human exposure. Endocrinology. 2006 Jun;147(6 Suppl):S56-69. ("Welshons 2006").

11  Sabrina Tavernise, F.D.A. Makes It Official: BPA Can't Be Used in Baby Bottles and Cups NYTimes, July 17, 2012.

12  Žalmanová, T., Hošková, K., Nevoral, J., Adámková, K., Kott, T., Šulc, M.,...& Petr, J. (2017). Bisphenol S negatively affects the meotic maturation of pig oocytes. Scientific reports, 7(1), 485. Campen, K. A., Kucharczyk, K. M., Bogin, B., Ehrlich, J. M., & Combelles, C. M. (2018). Spindle abnormalities and chromosome misalignment in bovine oocytes after exposure to low doses of bisphenol A or bisphenol S. Human Reproduction, 33(5), 895-904.

13  Lamb, J. D., M. S. Bloom, F. S. Vom Saal, J. A. Taylor, J. R. Sandler, and V. Y. Fujimoto. "Serum Bisphenol A (BPA) and reproductive outcomes in couples undergoing IVF." Fertil Steril. 2008; 90: S186.

14  Fujimoto VY, Kim D, vom Saal FS, Lamb JD, Taylor JA, Bloom MS. Serum unconjugated bisphenol A concentrations in women may adversely influence oocyte quality during in vitro fertilization. Fertil Steril. 2011 Apr;95(5):1816-9.

15  Mok-Lin E, Ehrlich S, Williams PL, Petrozza J, Wright DL, Calafat AM, Ye X, Hauser R. Urinary bisphenol A concentrations and ovarian response among women undergoing IVF. Int J Androl. 2010 Apr;33(2):385-93. ("Mok-Lin 2010").

16  Ehrlich S, Williams PL, Missmer SA, Flaws JA, Ye X, Calafat AM, Petrozza JC, Wright D, Hauser R. Urinary bisphenol A concentrations and early reproductive health outcomes among women undergoing IVF. Hum Reprod. 2012 Dec;27(12):3583-92

17  Ehrlich S, Williams PL, Missmer SA, Flaws JA, Berry KF, Calafat AM, Ye X, Petrozza JC, Wright D, Hauser R. Urinary bisphenol A concentrations and implantation failure among women undergoing in vitro fertilization. Environ Health Perspect. 2012 Jul;120(7):978-83.

18  Mínguez-Alarcón, L., Gaskins, A. J., Chiu, Y. H., Williams, P. L., Ehrlich, S., Chavarro, J. E.,...& Hauser, R. (2015). Urinary bisphenol A concentrations and association with in vitro fertilization outcomes among women from a fertility clinic. Human Reproduction, 30(9), 2120-2128.

19  Mínguez-Alarcón, L., Gaskins, A. J., Chiu, Y. H., Souter, I., Williams, P. L., Calafat, A. M.,...& EARTH Study team. (2016). Dietary folate intake and modification of the association of urinary bisphenol A

concentrations with in vitro fertilization outcomes among women from a fertility clinic. Reproductive Toxicology, 65, 104-112

20  Sugiura-Ogasawara M, Ozaki Y, Sonta S, Makino T, Suzumori K. Exposure to bisphenol A is associated with recurrent miscarriage. Hum Reprod. 2005 Aug;20(8):2325-9.

21  Shen, Y., Zheng, Y., Jiang, J., Liu, Y., Luo, X., Shen, Z., ... & Liang, H. (2015). Higher urinary bisphenol A concentration is associated with unexplained recurrent miscarriage risk: evidence from a case-control study in eastern China. PloS one, 10(5), e0127886.

22  R.B. Lathi et al, Maternal Serum Bisphenol-A (BPA) Level Is Positively Associated with Miscarriage Risk, O-6 , 69th Annual Meeting of the American Society for Reproductive Medicine, October 14, 2013.

23  Can A, Semiz O, Cinar O. Bisphenol-A induces cell cycle delay and alters centrosome and spindle microtubular organization in oocytes during meiosis. Mol Hum Reprod. 2005 Jun;11(6):389-96. ("Can 2005").
Lenie S, Cortvrindt R, Eichenlaub-Ritter U, Smitz J.Continuous exposure to bisphenol A during in vitro follicular development induces meiotic abnormalities. Mutat Res. 2008 Mar 12;651(1-2):71-81.
Xu J, Osuga Y, Yano T, Morita Y, Tang X, Fujiwara T, Takai Y, Matsumi H, Koga K, Taketani Y, Tsutsumi O. Bisphenol A induces apoptosis and G2-to-M arrest of ovarian granulosa cells. Biochem Biophys Res Commun. 2002 Mar 29;292(2):456-62.
Brieño-Enríquez MA, Robles P, Camats-Tarruella N, García-Cruz R, Roig I, Cabero L, Martínez F, Caldés MG. Human meiotic progression and recombination are affected by Bisphenol A exposure during in vitro human oocyte development. Hum Reprod. 2011 Oct;26(10):2807-18.

24  Li, Q., Davila, J., Kannan, A., Flaws, J. A., Bagchi, M. K., & Bagchi, I. C. (2016). Chronic exposure to Bisphenol A affects uterine function during early pregnancy in mice. Endocrinology, 157(5), 1764-1774. See also: Aldad, T. S., Rahmani, N., Leranth, C., & Taylor, H. S. (2011). Bisphenol-A exposure alters endometrial progesterone receptor expression in the nonhuman primate. Fertility and sterility, 96(1), 175-179.

25  Rudel RA, Gray JM, Engel CL, Rawsthorne TW, Dodson RE, Ackerman JM, Rizzo J, Nudelman JL, Brody JG. Food packaging and bisphenol A and bis(2-ethyhexyl) phthalate exposure: findings from a dietary intervention. Environ Health Perspect. 2011 Jul;119(7):914-20.

26 Campen, K. A., Kucharczyk, K. M., Bogin, B., Ehrlich, J. M., & Combelles, C. M. (2018). Spindle abnormalities and chromosome misalignment in bovine oocytes after exposure to low doses of bisphenol A or bisphenol S. Human Reproduction, 33(5), 895-904.
27 Fang, H., Wang, J., & Lynch, R. A. (2017). Migration of di (2-ethylhexyl) phthalate (DEHP) and di-n-butylphthalate (DBP) from polypropylene food containers. Food Control, 73, 1298-1302.
28 Lakind JS, Naiman DQ. Daily intake of bisphenol A and potential sources of exposure: 2005-2006 National Health and Nutrition Examination Survey. J Expo Sci Environ Epidemiol. 2011 May-Jun;21(3):272-9.
29 Bae B, Jeong JH, Lee SJ. The quantification and characterization of endocrine disruptor bisphenol-A leaching from epoxy resin. Water Sci Technol. 2002;46(11-12):381-7.
30 Geens T, Goeyens L, Covaci A. Are potential sources for human exposure to bisphenol-A overlooked? Int J Hyg Environ Health. 2011 Sep;214(5):339-47.
31 Biedermann S, Tschudin P, Grob K. Transfer of bisphenol A from thermal printer paper to the skin. Anal Bioanal Chem. 2010 Sep;398(1):571-6.
Zalko D, Jacques C, Duplan H, Bruel S, Perdu E.Viable skin efficiently absorbs and metabolizes bisphenol A.Chemosphere. 2011 Jan;82(3):424-30.
32 Lunder 2010, "BPA Coats Cash Register Receipts", http://www.ewg.org/bpa-in-store-receipts
33 vom Saal 2007.
34 Takahashi O, Oishi S. Disposition of orally administered 2,2-Bis(4-hydroxyphenyl)propane (Bisphenol A) in pregnant rats and the placental transfer to fetuses. Environ Health Perspect. 2000 Oct;108(10):931-5; Vom saal 2007.
35 E.g. Cabaton, Nicolas J., Perinaaz R. Wadia, Beverly S Rubin, Daniel Zalko, Cheryl M. Schaeberle, Michael H. Askenase, Jennifer L. Gadbois et al. "Perinatal exposure to environmentally relevant levels of bisphenol A decreases fertility and fecundity in CD-1 mice." Environmental health perspectives 119, no. 4 (2011): 547; Tharp, Andrew P., Maricel V. Maffini, Patricia A. Hunt, Catherine A. VandeVoort, Carlos Sonnenschein, and Ana M. Soto. "Bisphenol A alters the development of the rhesus monkey mammary gland." *Proceedings of the National Academy of Sciences* 109, no. 21 (2012): 8190-8195; Tian, Yu-Hua, Joung-Hee Baek, Seok-Yong Lee, and Choon-Gon Jang. "Prenatal and postnatal exposure to

bisphenol a induces anxiolytic behaviors and cognitive deficits in mice." *Synapse* 64, no. 6 (2010): 432-439; Jang, Young Jung, Hee Ra Park, Tae Hyung Kim, Wook-Jin Yang, Jong-Joo Lee, Seon Young Choi, Shin Bi Oh et al. "High dose bisphenol A impairs hippocampal neurogenesis in female mice across generations." *Toxicology* (2012). Somm, Emmanuel, Valérie M. Schwitzgebel, Audrey Toulotte, Christopher R. Cederroth, Christophe Combescure, Serge Nef, Michel L. Aubert, and Petra S. Hüppi. "Perinatal exposure to bisphenol a alters early adipogenesis in the rat." *Environmental Health Perspectives* 117, no. 10 (2009): 1549. Braun, Joe M., Amy E. Kalkbrenner, Antonia M. Calafat, Kimberly Yolton, Xiaoyun Ye, Kim N. Dietrich, and Bruce P. Lanphear. "Impact of early-life bisphenol A exposure on behavior and executive function in children." *Pediatrics* 128, no. 5 (2011): 873-882.

36 Braun JM, Yolton K, Dietrich KN, Hornung R, Ye X, Calafat AM, Lanphear BP. Prenatal bisphenol A exposure and early childhood behavior. Environ Health Perspect. 2009 Dec;117(12):1945-52.

## Chapter 3: Phthalates

1 Meeker JD, Sathyanarayana S, Swan SH.Phthalates and other additives in plastics: human exposure and associated health outcomes. Philos Trans R Soc Lond B Biol Sci. 2009 Jul 27;364(1526):2097-113.

2 Hauser R, Calafat AM. Phthalates and human health. Occup Environ Med. 2005 Nov;62(11):806-18.;

3 Directive 2005/84/EC of the European Parliament and of the Council of 14 December 2005.

4 U.S. Department of Health and Human Services, Food and Drug Administration, Center for Drug Evaluation and Research (CDER). Guidance for Industry: Limiting the Use of Certain Phthalates as Excipients in CDER-Regulated Products, December 2012.

5 David Byrne, EU Commissioner for Consumer Protection and Health, November 10th, 1999. http://europa.eu/rapid/press-release_IP-99-829_en.htm?locale=FR

6 Interview with EurActiv, 05/09/2012. http://www.euractiv.com/sustainability/us-scientist-routes-exposure-end-interview-512402

7 Berman T, Hochner-Celnikier D, Calafat AM, Needham LL, Amitai Y, Wormser U, et al. Phthalate exposure among pregnant women in Jerusalem, Israel: results of a pilot study. Environ Int. 2009;35:353–7.

8 Göen T, Dobler L, Koschorreck J, Müller J, Wiesmüller GA, Drexler H, Kolossa-Gehring M. Trends of the internal phthalate

exposure of young adults in Germany—follow-up of a retrospective human biomonitoring study. Int J Hyg Environ Health. 2011 Dec;215(1):36-45.

Silva MJ, Barr DB, Reidy JA, Malek NA, Hodge CC, Caudill SP, Brock JW, Needham LL, Calafat AM. Urinary levels of seven phthalate metabolites in the U.S. population from the National Health and Nutrition Examination Survey (NHANES) 1999-2000. Environ Health Perspect. 2004 Mar;112(3):331-8.

Lin S, Ku HY, Su PH, Chen JW, Huang PC, Angerer J, Wang SL. Phthalate exposure in pregnant women and their children in central Taiwan. Chemosphere. 2011 Feb;82(7):947-55.

9   Davis BJ, Maronpot RR, Heindel JJ.Di-(2-ethylhexyl) phthalate suppresses estradiol and ovulation in cycling rats.Toxicol Appl Pharmacol. 1994 Oct;128(2):216-23.

10  Anas MK, Suzuki C, Yoshioka K, Iwamura S. Effect of mono-(2-ethylhexyl) phthalate on bovine oocyte maturation in vitro. Reprod Toxicol. 2003 May-Jun;17(3):305-10; Ambruosi B, Uranio MF, Sardanelli AM, Pocar P, Martino NA, Paternoster MS, Amati F, Dell'Aquila ME. In vitro acute exposure to DEHP affects oocyte meiotic maturation, energy and oxidative stress parameters in a large animal model. PLoS One. 2011;6(11):e27452; Grossman D, Kalo D, Gendelman M, Roth Z.Effect of di-(2-ethylhexyl) phthalate and mono-(2-ethylhexyl) phthalate on in vitro developmental competence of bovine oocytes. Cell Biol Toxicol. 2012 Dec;28(6):383-96. ("Grossman 2012"). Gupta RK, Singh JM, Leslie TC, Meachum S, Flaws JA, Yao HH. Di-(2-ethylhexyl) phthalate and mono-(2-ethylhexyl) phthalate inhibit growth and reduce estradiol levels of antral follicles in vitro. Toxicol Appl Pharmacol. 2010 Jan 15;242(2):224-30. ("Gupta 2010").

11  Huang XF, Li Y, Gu YH, Liu M, Xu Y, Yuan Y, Sun F, Zhang HQ, Shi HJ. The effects of Di-(2-ethylhexyl)-phthalate exposure on fertilization and embryonic development in vitro and testicular genomic mutation in vivo. PLoS One. 2012;7(11):e50465. Pant N, Pant A, Shukla M, Mathur N, Gupta Y, Saxena D. Environmental and experimental exposure of phthalate esters: the toxicological consequence on human sperm. Hum Exp Toxicol. 2011 Jun;30(6):507-14.

12  Duty S. M., Singh N. P., Silva M. J., Barr D. B., Brock J. W., Ryan L., Herrick R. F., Christiani D. C., Hauser R. 2003b. The relationship between environmental exposures to phthalates and DNA damage in human sperm using the neutral comet assay. Environ. Health Perspect. 111, 1164–1169. ("In conclusion, this

study represents the first human data to demonstrate that urinary MEP, at environmental levels, is associated with increased DNA damage in sperm.")

13  Gupta 2010; Grossman 2012

14  Gupta 2010; Grossman 2012.
   Reinsberg J, Wegener-Toper P, van der Ven K, van der Ven H, Klingmueller D. Effect of mono-(2-ethylhexyl) phthalate on steroid production of human granulosa cells. Toxicol Appl Pharmacol. 2009 Aug 15;239(1):116-23.
   Lenie S, Smitz J. Steroidogenesis-disrupting compounds can be effectively studied for major fertility-related endpoints using in vitro cultured mouse follicles. Toxicol Lett. 2009 Mar 28;185(3):143-52
   Dalman A, Eimani H, Sepehri H, Ashtiani SK, Valojerdi MR, Eftekhari-Yazdi P, Shahverdi A. Effect of mono-(2-ethylhexyl) phthalate (MEHP) on resumption of meiosis, in vitro maturation and embryo development of immature mouse oocytes. Biofactors. 2008;33(2):149-55. ("Dalman 2008").

15  Hong YC, Park EY, Park MS, Ko JA, Oh SY, Kim H, Lee KH, Leem JH, Ha EH. Community level exposure to chemicals and oxidative stress in adult population. Toxicol. Lett. 2009;184(2):139–144; Ferguson KK, Loch-Caruso R, Meeker JD.Urinary phthalate metabolites in relation to biomarkers of inflammation and oxidative stress: NHANES 1999-2006.Environ Res. 2011 Jul;111(5):718-26. ("Ferguson 2011").

16  Agarwal A, Gupta S, Sekhon L, Shah R. Redox considerations in female reproductive function and assisted reproduction: from molecular mechanisms to health implications. Antioxid Redox Signal. 2008 Aug;10(8):1375-403.
   Zhang X, Wu XQ, Lu S, Guo YL, Ma X.Deficit of mitochondria-derived ATP during oxidative stress impairs mouse MII oocyte spindles.Cell Res. 2006 Oct;16(10):841-50. , Lim and Lauderer 2010 in Wang)

17  Agarwal A, Aponte-Mellado A, Premkumar BJ, Shaman A, Gupta S. The effects of oxidative stress on female reproduction: a review. Reprod Biol Endocrinol. 2012 Jun 29;10:49
   Ruder EH, Hartman TJ, Goldman MB. Impact of oxidative stress on female fertility. Curr Opin Obstet Gynecol. 2009 Jun;21(3):219-22.
   Al-Gubory KH, Fowler PA, Garrel C. The roles of cellular reactive oxygen species, oxidative stress and antioxidants in pregnancy outcomes. Int J Biochem Cell Biol. 2010; 42:1634–1650.

18  Ferguson 2011.

19  Liu K, Lehmann KP, Sar M, Young SS, Gaido KW. Gene expression profiling following in utero exposure to phthalate esters reveals new gene targets in the etiology of testicular dysgenesis. Biol Reprod. 2005; 73:180–192.
Botelho GG, Bufalo AC, Boareto AC, Muller JC, Morais RN, Martino-Andrade AJ, Lemos KR, Dalsenter PR. Vitamin C and resveratrol supplementation to rat dams treated with di(2-ethylhexyl)phthalate: impact on reproductive and oxidative stress end points in male offspring. Arch Environ Contam Toxicol. 2009; 57:785–793
Erkekoglu P, Rachidi W, Yuzugullu OG, Giray B, Favier A, Ozturk M, Hincal F. Evaluation of cytotoxicity and oxidative DNA damaging effects of di(2-ethylhexyl)-phthalate (DEHP) and mono(2-ethylhexyl)-phthalate (MEHP) on MA-10 Leydig cells and protection by selenium. Toxicol Appl Pharmacol. 2010; 248:52–62.

20  Wang W, Craig ZR, Basavarajappa MS, Gupta RK, Flaws JA. Di (2-ethylhexyl) phthalate inhibits growth of mouse ovarian antral follicles through an oxidative stress pathway. Toxicol Appl Pharmacol. 2012 Jan 15;258(2):288-95. ("Wang 2012"); C.f. Ambruosi 2011.

21  Hauser R, Gaskins AJ, Souter I, Smith KW, Dodge LE, Ehrlich S, Meeker JD, Calafat AM, Williams PL, EARTH Study Team. Urinary phthalate metabolite concentrations and reproductive outcomes among women undergoing in vitro fertilization: results from the EARTH study. Environmental Health Perspectives. 2016 Jun 1;124(6);831

22  Cobellis L, Latini G, De Felice C, Razzi S, Paris I, Ruggieri F, et al. High plasma concentrations of di-(2-ethylhexyl)-phthalate in women with endometriosis. Hum Reprod. 2003;18:1512–5.
Reddy BS, Rozati R, Reddy BV, Raman NV. Association of phthalate esters with endometriosis in Indian women. Bjog. 2006;113:515–20.

23  Kim SH, Chun S, Jang JY, Chae HD, Kim CH, Kang BM. Increased plasma levels of phthalate esters in women with advanced-stage endometriosis: a prospective case-control study. Fertil Steril. 2011 Jan;95(1):357-9.
Reddy BS, Rozati R, Reddy S, Kodampur S, Reddy P, Reddy R. High plasma concentrations of polychlorinated biphenyls and phthalate esters in women with endometriosis: a prospective case control study. Fertil Steril. 2006 Mar;85(3):775-9;
Weuve J, Hauser R, Calafat AM, Missmer SA, Wise LA. Association of exposure to phthalates with endometriosis and

uterine leiomyomata: findings from NHANES, 1999-2004. Environ Health Perspect. 2010 Jun;118(6):825-32.

24  Buck Louis GM, Peterson CM, Chen Z, Croughan M, Sundaram R, Stanford J, Varner MW, Kennedy A, Giudice L, Fujimoto VY, Sun L, Wang L, Guo Y, Kannan K.Bisphenol A and phthalates and endometriosis: the Endometriosis: Natural History, Diagnosis and Outcomes Study .Fertil Steril. 2013 Jul;100(1):162-9.e1-2.

25  Toft G, Jönsson BA, Lindh CH, Jensen TK, Hjollund NH, Vested A, Bonde JP. Association between pregnancy loss and urinary phthalate levels around the time of conception. Environ Health Perspect. 2012 Mar;120(3):458-63.

26  Koch, H. M., Lorber, M., Christensen, K. L., Pälmke, C., Koslitz, S., & Brüning, T. (2013). Identifying sources of phthalate exposure with human biomonitoring: results of a 48 h fasting study with urine collection and personal activity patterns. International journal of hygiene and environmental health, 216(6), 672-681.

27  Zota, A. R., Phillips, C. A., & Mitro, S. D. (2016). Recent fast food consumption and bisphenol A and phthalates exposures among the US population in NHANES, 2003–2010. Environmental health perspectives, 124(10), 1521.

28  Rudel RA, Gray JM, Engel CL, Rawsthorne TW, Dodson RE, Ackerman JM, Rizzo J, Nudelman JL, Brody JG. Food packaging and bisphenol A and bis(2-ethyhexyl) phthalate exposure: findings from a dietary intervention. Environ Health Perspect. 2011 Jul;119(7):914-20.

29  Cao, X. L., Zhao, W., Churchill, R., & Hilts, C. (2014). Occurrence of di-(2-ethylhexyl) adipate and phthalate plasticizers in samples of meat, fish, and cheese and their packaging films. Journal of food protection, 77(4), 610-620.

30  Van Holderbeke, M., Geerts, L., Vanermen, G., Servaes, K., Sioen, I., De Henauw, S., & Fierens, T. (2014). Determination of contamination pathways of phthalates in food products sold on the Belgian market. Environmental research, 134, 345-352.

31  Lin, J., Chen, W., Zhu, H., & Wang, C. (2015). Determination of free and total phthalates in commercial whole milk products in different packaging materials by gas chromatography-mass spectrometry. Journal of dairy science, 98(12), 8278-8284.

32  Montuori P, Jover E, Morgantini M, Bayona JM, Triassi M. Assessing human exposure to phthalic acid and phthalate esters from mineral water stored in polyethylene terephthalate and glass bottles. Food Add Contamin. 2008;25(4):511–518;

Sax L. Polyethylene terephthalate may yield endocrine disruptors. Environ Health Perspect. 2010;118:445–8; Farhoodi M, Emam-Djomeh Z, Ehsani MR, Oromiehie A. Effect of environmental conditions on the migration of di(2-ethylhexyl)phthalate from PET bottles into yogurt drinks: influence of time, temperature, and food simulant. Arabian J Sci Eng. 2008;33(2):279–287.

33 Wittassek M, Koch HM, Angerer J, Bruning T. Assessing exposure to phthalates – the human biomonitoring approach. Mol Nutr Food Res. 2011;55:7–31

34 Koniecki D, Wang R, Moody RP, Zhu J.Phthalates in cosmetic and personal care products: concentrations and possible dermal exposure.Environ Res. 2011 Apr;111(3):329-36. ("Koniecki 2011"). Janjua NR, Mortensen GK, Andersson AM, Kongshoj B, Skakkebaek NE, Wulf HC.Systemic uptake of diethyl phthalate, dibutyl phthalate, and butyl paraben following whole-body topical application and reproductive and thyroid hormone levels in humans. Environ Sci Technol. 2007 Aug 1;41(15):5564-70.

35 Koniecki 2011.

36 Plenge-Bönig A, Karmaus W. Exposure to toluene in the printing industry is associated with subfecundity in women but not in men. Occup Environ Med. 1999 Jul;56(7):443-8. Svensson BG, Nise G, Erfurth EM, Nilsson A, Skerfving S. Hormone status in occupational toluene exposure. Am J Ind Med. 1992;22(1):99–107. Ng TP, Foo SC, Yoong T Risk of spontaneous abortion in workers exposed to toluene. Br J Ind Med. 1992 Nov;49(11):804–808; Taskinen HK, Kyyrönen P, Sallmén M, Virtanen SV, Liukkonen TA, Huida O, Lindbohm ML, Anttila A. Reduced fertility among female wood workers exposed to formaldehyde. Am J Ind Med. 1999 Jul;36(1):206-12.

37 Lindbohm ML, Hemminki K, Bonhomme MG, Anttila A, Rantala K, Heikkila P, Rosenberg MJ. Effects of paternal occupational exposure on spontaneous abortions. American Journal of Public Health. 1991;81:1029–1033 Saurel-Cubizolles MJ, Hays M, Estryn-Behar M. Work in operating rooms and pregnancy outcome among nurses. Int Arch Occup Environ Health. 1994;66:235–241. John EM, Savitz DA, Shy CM. Spontaneous abortions among cosmetologists. Epidemiology. 1994;5:147–155.

38 Koniecki 2011.

39 Smith KW, Souter I, Dimitriadis I, Ehrlich S, Williams PL, Calafat AM, Hauser R. Urinary paraben concentrations and ovarian aging

among women from a fertility center. Environ Health Perspect 2013 Aug;121:1299–1305.

40  Latini G, et al. In utero exposure to di-(2-ethylhexyl)phthalate and duration of human pregnancy. Environmental Health Perspectives. 2003;111:1783–1785.

Meeker JD, Hu H, Cantonwine DE, Lamadrid-Figueroa H, Calafat AM, Ettinger AS, Hernandez-Avila M, Loch-Caruso R, Téllez-Rojo MM. Urinary phthalate metabolites in relation to preterm birth in Mexico city. Environ. Health Perspect. 2009;117(10):1587–1592.

Whyatt RM, Adibi JJ, Calafat AM, Camann DE, Rauh V, Bhat HK, Perera FP, Andrews H, Just AC, Hoepner L, Tang D, Hauser R. Prenatal di(2-ethylhexyl) phthalate exposure and length of gestation among an inner-city cohort. Pediatrics. 2009;124(6):e1213–e1220.

Swan SH, Main KM, Liu F, Stewart SL, Kruse RL, Calafat AM, Mao CS, Redmon JB, Ternand CL, Sullivan S, Teague JL; Study for Future Families Research Team.Decrease in anogenital distance among male infants with prenatal phthalateexposure. Environ Health Perspect. 2005 Aug;113(8):1056-61. Erratum in: Environ Health Perspect. 2005 Sep;113(9):A583. ("Swan 2005").

Swan SH. Environmental phthalate exposure in relation to reproductive outcomes and other health endpoints in humans. Environ Res. 2008 Oct; 108(2):177-84

41  Bornehag, C. G., Lindh, C., Reichenberg, A., Wikström, S., Hallerback, M. U., Evans, S. F., ... & Swan, S. H. (2018). Association of prenatal phthalate exposure with language development in early childhood. JAMA pediatrics, 172(12), 1169-1176.

42  http://www.ewg.org/research/dirty-dozen-list-endocrine-disruptors

43  http://www.ewg.org/report/ewgs-water-filter-buying-guide

44  Messerlian, C., Williams, P. L., Mínguez-Alarcón, L., Carignan, C. C., Ford, J. B., Butt, C. M., ... & EARTH Study Team. (2018). Organophosphate flame-retardant metabolite concentrations and pregnancy loss among women conceiving with assisted reproductive technology. Fertility and sterility, 110(6), 1137-1144.

Small, C. M., Murray, D., Terrell, M. L., & Marcus, M. (2011). Reproductive outcomes among women exposed to a brominated flame retardant in utero. Archives of environmental & occupational health, 66(4), 201-208.

45  Melin, V. E., Potineni, H., Hunt, P., Griswold, J., Siems, B., Werre, S. R., & Hrubec, T. C. (2014). Exposure to common quaternary ammonium disinfectants decreases fertility in mice. Reproductive toxicology, 50, 163-170.

46  Interview with EurActiv, 05/09/2012.
http://www.euractiv.com/sustainability/us-scientist-routes-
exposure-end-interview-512402

## Chapter 4: Unexpected Obstacles to Fertility

1  Aleyasin A, Hosseini MA, Mahdavi A, Safdarian L, Fallahi P,
Mohajeri MR, Abbasi M, Esfahani F.Predictive value of the
level of vitamin D in follicular fluid on the outcome of assisted
reproductive technology.Eur J Obstet Gynecol Reprod Biol. 2011
Nov;159(1):132-7.
Anifandis GM, Dafopoulos K, Messini CI, Chalvatzas N, Liakos
N, Pournaras S, Messinis IE. Prognostic value of follicular fluid
25-OH vitamin D and glucose levels in the IVF outcome. Reprod
Biol Endocrinol. 2010 Jul 28;8:91.
2  Rudick B, Ingles S, Chung K, Stanczyk F, Paulson R, Bendikson K.
Characterizing the influence of vitamin D levels on IVF outcomes.
Hum Reprod. 2012 Nov;27(11):3321-7. ("Rudick 2012").
3  Ozkan S, Jindal S, Greenseid K, Shu J, Zeitlian G, Hickmon C, Pal
L. Replete vitamin D stores predict reproductive success following
in vitro fertilization. Fertil Steril. 2010 Sep;94(4):1314-9.
4  Firouzabadi RD, Rahmani E, Rahsepar M, Firouzabadi MM. Value
of follicular fluid vitamin D in predicting the pregnancy rate in an
IVF program. Arch Gynecol Obstet. 2014 Jan;289(1):201 6
5  Ruddick 2012). Rudick B, Ingles S, Chung K, Stanczyk F, Paulson
R, Bendikson K. Characterizing the influence of vitamin D levels
on IVF outcomes. Hum Reprod. 2012 Nov;27(11):3321-7.
6  Luk 2012.
7  Luk J, Torrealday S, Neal Perry G, Pal L. Relevance of vitamin D in
reproduction. Hum Reprod. 2012 Oct;27(10):3015-27 ("Luk 2012").
8  Li HW, Brereton RE, Anderson RA, Wallace AM, Ho CK. Vitamin
D deficiency is common and associated with metabolic risk factors
in patients with polycystic ovary syndrome. Metabolism. 2011
Oct;60(10):1475-81
Wehr E, Pilz S, Schweighofer N, Giuliani A, Kopera D, Pieber
TR, Obermayer-Pietsch B. Association of hypovitaminosis D
with metabolic disturbances in polycystic ovary syndrome. Eur J
Endocrinol. 2009 Oct;161(4):575-82.
Wehr E, Pieber TR, Obermayer-Pietsch B. Effect of vitamin D3
treatment on glucose metabolism and menstrual frequency in
polycystic ovary syndrome women: a pilot study. J Endocrinol
Invest. 2011 Nov;34(10):757-63

Miyashita, M., Koga, K., Izumi, G., Sue, F., Makabe, T., Taguchi, A.,...& Hirata, T. (2016). Effects of 1, 25-dihydroxy vitamin D3 on endometriosis. The Journal of Clinical Endocrinology & Metabolism, 101(6), 2371-2379.

Ciavattini, A., Serri, M., Delli Carpini, G., Morini, S., & Clemente, N. (2017). Ovarian endometriosis and vitamin D serum levels. Gynecological Endocrinology, 33(2), 164-167.

9  Masbou, A. K., Kramer, Y., Taveras, D., McCulloh, D. H., & Grifo, J. A. (2018). Vitamin D deficiency at time of frozen embryo transfer is associated with increased miscarriage rate but does not impact folliculogenesis. Fertility and Sterility, 109(3), e37-e38.

Mumford, S. L., Garbose, R. A., Kim, K., Kissell, K., Kuhr, D. L., Omosigho, U. R.,...& Plowden, T. C. (2018). Association of preconception serum 25-hydroxyvitamin D concentrations with livebirth and pregnancy loss: a prospective cohort study. The Lancet Diabetes & Endocrinology.

10  Ota, K., Dambaeva, S., Han, A. R., Beaman, K., Gilman-Sachs, A., & Kwak-Kim, J. (2013). Vitamin D deficiency may be a risk factor for recurrent pregnancy losses by increasing cellular immunity and autoimmunity. Human reproduction, 29(2), 208-219.

Chen, X., Yin, B., Lian, R. C., Zhang, T., Zhang, H. Z., Diao, L. H.,...& Zeng, Y. (2016). Modulatory effects of vitamin D on peripheral cellular immunity in patients with recurrent miscarriage. American Journal of Reproductive Immunology, 76(6), 432-438.

11  Looker AC, Pfeiffer CM, Lacher DA, Schleicher RL, Picciano MF, Yetley EA. Serum 25-hydroxyvitamin D status of the US population: 1988-1994 compared with 2000-2004. Am J Clin Nutr. 2008 Dec;88(6):1519-27 ("Looker 2008");

Nesby-O'Dell S, Scanlon KS, Cogswell ME, Gillespie C, Hollis BW, Looker AC, Allen C, Doughertly C, Gunter EW, Bowman BA. Hypovitaminosis D prevalence and determinants among African American and white women of reproductive age: third National Health and Nutrition Examination Survey, 1988-1994. Am J Clin Nutr. 2002 Jul;76(1):187-92

12  Ginde, A. A., Sullivan, A. F., Mansbach, J. M., & Camargo Jr, C. A. (2010). Vitamin D insufficiency in pregnant and nonpregnant women of childbearing age in the United States. American journal of obstetrics and gynecology, 202(5), 436-e1.

Haq, A., Svobodová, J., Imran, S., Stanford, C., & Razzaque, M. S. (2016). Vitamin D deficiency: A single centre analysis of patients from 136 countries. The Journal of steroid biochemistry and molecular biology, 164, 209-213.

13   Hollis, B. W., & Wagner, C. L. (2017). New insights into the vitamin D requirements during pregnancy. Bone research, 5, 17030.

14   Smolders, J., Peelen, E., Thewissen, M., Tervaert, J. W. C., Menheere, P., Hupperts, R., & Damoiseaux, J. (2010). Safety and T cell modulating effects of high dose vitamin D3 supplementation in multiple sclerosis. PLoS One, 5(12), e15235.

15   Razavi, M., Jamilian, M., Karamali, M., Bahmani, F., Aghadavod, E., & Asemi, Z. (2016). The effects of vitamin DK-calcium co-supplementation on endocrine, inflammation, and oxidative stress biomarkers in vitamin D-deficient women with polycystic ovary syndrome: a randomized, double-blind, placebo-controlled trial. Hormone and Metabolic Research, 48(07), 446-451.

16   Grossmann RE, Tangpricha V. Evaluation of vehicle substances on vitamin D bioavailability: a systematic review. Mol Nutr Food Res. 2010 Aug;54(8):1055-61; Raimundo FV, Faulhaber GA, Menegatti PK, Marques Lda S, Furlanetto TW. Effect of High- versus Low-Fat Meal on Serum 25-Hydroxyvitamin D Levels after a Single Oral Dose of Vitamin D: A Single-Blind, Parallel, Randomized Trial. Int J Endocrinol. 2011;2011:809069.

17   Stagnaro-Green A, Roman SH, Cobin RH, el-Harazy E, Alvarez-Marfany M, Davies TF. Detection of at-risk pregnancy by means of highly sensitive assays for thyroid autoantibodies. JAMA. 1990 Sep 19;264(11):1422-5 ("Stagnaro-Green 1990"), Thangaratinam S, Tan A, Knox E, Kilby MD, Franklyn J, Coomarasamy A. Association between thyroid autoantibodies and miscarriage and preterm birth: meta-analysis of evidence. BMJ. 2011 May 9;342:d2616. ("Thangaratinam 2011").

18   Stagnaro-Green 1990.

19   Stagnaro-Green A. Thyroid antibodies and miscarriage: where are we at a generation later? J Thyroid Res. 2011; 2011:841949.

20   Ghafoor F, Mansoor M, Malik T, Malik MS, Khan AU, Edwards R, Akhtar W. Role of thyroid peroxidase antibodies in the outcome of pregnancy. J Coll Physicians Surg Pak. 2006 Jul;16(7):468-71.

21   Pratt DE, Kaberlein G, Dudkiewicz A, Karande V, Gleicher N. The association of antithyroid antibodies in euthyroid nonpregnant women with recurrent first trimester abortions in the next pregnancy. Fertil Steril. 1993 Dec;60(6):1001-5; Bussen S, Steck T. Thyroid autoantibodies in euthyroid non-pregnant women with recurrent spontaneous abortions. Hum Reprod. 1995 Nov;10(11):2938-40; Dendrinos S, Papasteriades C, Tarassi K,

Christodoulakos G, Prasinos G, Creatsas G. Thyroid autoimmunity in patients with recurrent spontaneous miscarriages. Gynecol Endocrinol. 2000 Aug;14(4):270-4.

22 Toulis KA, Goulis DG, Venetis CA, Kolibianakis EM, Negro R, Tarlatzis BC, Papadimas I. Risk of spontaneous miscarriage in euthyroid women with thyroid autoimmunity undergoing IVF: a meta-analysis. Eur J Endocrinol. 2010 Apr;162(4):643-52; Prummel MF, Wiersinga WM. Thyroid autoimmunity and miscarriage. Eur J Endocrinol. 2004 Jun;150(6):751-5; Thangaratinam 2011

23 Negro R, Schwartz A, Gismondi R, Tinelli A, Mangieri T, Stagnaro-Green A. Increased pregnancy loss rate in thyroid antibody negative women with TSH levels between 2.5 and 5.0 in the first trimester of pregnancy. J Clin Endocrinol Metab. 2010 Sep;95(9):E44-8. ("Negro 2010").

24 Negro 2010.

25 Negro R, Formoso G, Mangieri T, Pezzarossa A, Dazzi D, Hassan H. Levothyroxine treatment in euthyroid pregnant women with autoimmune thyroid disease: effects on obstetrical complications. J Clin Endocrinol Metab. 2006 Jul;91(7):2587-91.

26 Kim CH, Ahn JW, Kang SP, Kim SH, Chae HD, Kang BM. Effect of levothyroxine treatment on in vitro fertilization and pregnancy outcome in infertile women with subclinical hypothyroidism undergoing in vitro fertilization/intracytoplasmic sperm injection. Fertil Steril. 2011 Apr;95(5):1650-4. ("Kim 2011").

27 Abalovich M, Mitelberg L, Allami C, Gutierrez S, Alcaraz G, Otero P, Levalle O. Subclinical hypothyroidism and thyroid autoimmunity in women with infertility. Gynecol Endocrinol. 2007 May;23(5):279-83. ("Abalovich 2007").

28 Eldar-Geva T, Shoham M, Rösler A, Margalioth EJ, Livne K, Meirow D. Subclinical hypothyroidism in infertile women: the importance of continuous monitoring and the role of the thyrotropin-releasing hormone stimulation test. Gynecol Endocrinol. 2007 Jun;23(6):332-7.

29 Abalovich 2007

30 Kim 2011.

31 Janssen OE, Mehlmauer N, Hahn S, Offner AH, Gärtner R. High prevalence of autoimmune thyroiditis in patients with polycystic ovary syndrome. Eur J Endocrinol. 2004 Mar;150(3):363-9. Sinha U, Sinharay K, Saha S, Longkumer TA, Baul SN, Pal SK. Thyroid disorders in polycystic ovarian syndrome subjects: A

tertiary hospital based cross-sectional study from Eastern India .Indian J Endocrinol Metab. 2013 Mar;17(2):304-9.

32 Myers, A, (2016), *The Thyroid Connection*. Little, Brown. P. 119.

33 Fasano A, Catassi C. Current Approaches to Diagnosis and Treatment of Celiac Disease: An Evolving Spectrum. Gastroenterology, 2001;120:636-651.

34 Kaukinen K, Maki M, Collin P. Immunohistochemical features in antiendomysium positive patients with normal villous architecture. Am J Gastroenterol, 2006;101(3):675-676; Kumar V. American Celiac Society, Nov.9,1999.

35 Pellicano R., Astegiano M., Bruno M., Fagoonee S., Rizzetto M.. Women and celiac disease: association with unexplained infertility. Minerva Med, 2007;98:217-219. ("Pellicano 2007").

36 Ferguson R, Holmes GK, Cooke WT. Coeliac disease, fertility, and pregnancy. Scand J Gastroenterol, 1982;17:65–68.

37 Choi JM, Lebwohl B, Wang J, Lee SK, Murray JA, Sauer MV, Green PH. Increased prevalence of celiac disease in patients with unexplained infertility in the United States.J Reprod Med. 2011 May-Jun;56(5-6):199-203. ("Choi 2011");
Jackson, J. E., Rosen, M., McLean, T., Moro, J., Croughan, M., & Cedars, M. I. (2008). Prevalence of celiac disease in a cohort of women with unexplained infertility. Fertility and sterility, 89(4), 1002-1004.
Kumar A, Meena M, Begum N, Kumar N, Gupta RK, Aggarwal S, Prasad S, Batra S. Latent celiac disease in reproductive performance of women. Fertil Steril. 2011 Mar 1;95(3):922-7; Machado AP, Silva LR, Zausner B, Oliveira Jde A, Diniz DR, de Oliveira J. Undiagnosed celiac disease in women with infertility. J Reprod Med. 2013 Jan-Feb;58(1-2):61-6; Pellicano 2007.

38 Choi 2011.

39 Singh, P., Arora, S., Lal, S., Strand, T. A., & Makharia, G. K. (2016). Celiac Disease in Women With Infertility. Journal of clinical gastroenterology, 50(1), 33-39.

40 Juneau, C. R., Marin, D., Scott, K., Morin, S. J., Neal, S. A., Juneau, J., & Scott, R. T. (2017). Cares trial (celiac disease and reproductive effects): celiac disease is not more common in patients undergoing IVF and outcomes are not compromised in affected patients. Fertility and Sterility, 108(3), e33-e34.

41 Ciacci C, Cirillo M, Auriemma G, Di Dato G, Sabbatini F, Mazzacca G. Celiac disease and pregnancy outcome. Am J Gastroenterol, 1996;91(4):718-722.

42 Pellicano 2007.

43 Dickey W, Ward M, Whittle CR, Kelly MT, Pentieva K, Horigan G, Patton S, McNulty H. Homocysteine and related B-vitamin status in coeliac disease: Effects of gluten exclusion and histological recovery. Scand J Gastroenterol. 2008;43(6):682-8. ("Dickey 2008"). Ocal 2012. Ocal P, Ersoylu B, Cepni I, Guralp O, Atakul N, Irez T, Idil M.The association between homocysteine in the follicular fluid with embryo quality and pregnancy rate in assisted reproductive techniques. J Assist Reprod Genet. 2012 Apr;29(4):299-304.

44 Dickey 2008.

45 Hallert C, Grant C, Grehn S, Grännö C, Hultén S, Midhagen G, Ström M, Svensson H, Valdimarsson T.Evidence of poor vitamin status in coeliac patients on a gluten-free diet for 10 years. Aliment Pharmacol Ther. 2002 Jul;16(7):1333-9.

46 Hallert C, Svensson M, Tholstrup J, Hultberg B.Clinical trial: B vitamins improve health in patients with coeliac disease living on a gluten-free diet. Aliment Pharmacol Ther. 2009 Apr 15;29(8):811-6.

47 La Villa G, Pantaleo P, Tarquini R, Cirami L, Perfetto F, Mancuso F, Laffi G. Multiple immune disorders in unrecognized celiac disease: a case report. World J Gastroenterol, 2003;9(6): 1377-1380. ("La Villa 2003").

48 La Villa 2003.

49 Bast 2009.

50 Ide M, Papapanou PN. Epidemiology of association between maternal periodontal disease and adverse pregnancy outcomes—systematic review. J Periodontol. 2013 Apr;84(4 Suppl):S181-94. Vogt M, Sallum AW, Cecatti JG, Morais SS. Periodontal disease and some adverse perinatal outcomes in a cohort of low risk pregnant women. Reprod Health. 2010 Nov 3;7:29 Offenbacher S, Beck JD. Periodontitis: a potential risk factor for spontaneous preterm birth. Compend. Contin. Educ. Dent.22(2 Spec No),17–20 (2001). Shub A, Wong C, Jennings B, Swain JR, Newnham JP. Maternal periodontal disease and perinatal mortality. Aust N Z J Obstet Gynaecol 2009;49:130-136.

51 Jeffcoat MK, Geurs NC, Reddy MS, Cliver SP, Goldenberg RL, Hauth JC. Periodontal infection and preterm birth: results of a prospective study. J Am Dent Assoc. 2001 Jul;132(7):875-80

52 Farrell S, Ide M, Wilson RF. The relationship between maternal periodontitis, adverse pregnancy outcome and miscarriage in never smokers. J Clin Periodontol. 2006 Feb;33(2):115-20.

53 Madianos PN, Bobetsis YA, Offenbacher S.Adverse pregnancy outcomes (APOs) and

periodontal disease: pathogenic mechanisms.J Periodontol. 2013 Apr;84(4 Suppl):S170-80.

54 Hart R, Doherty DA, Pennell CE, Newnham IA, Newnham JP. Periodontal disease: a potential modifiable risk factor limiting conception. Hum Reprod. 2012 May;27(5):1332-42.

55 Newnham JP, Newnham IA, Ball CM, Wright M, Pennell CE, Swain J, Doherty DA. Treatment of periodontal disease during pregnancy: a randomized controlled trial. Obstet Gynecol 2009;114:1239-1248.

## Chapter 5: Prenatal Multivitamins

1 CDC, ten great public health achievements- United States, 2001-2010. Morb Mortal Wkly Rep 2011: 60-619-23.

2 Prevention of neural tube defects: results of the Medical Research Council Vitamin Study MRC Vitamin Study Research Group. Lancet. 1991 Jul 20;338(8760):131-7.

3 Smithells RW, Sheppard S, Schorah CJ, Seller MJ, Nevin NC, Harris R, Read AP, Fielding DW.Apparent prevention of neural tube defects by periconceptional vitamin supplementation. 1981.Int J Epidemiol. 2011 Oct;40(5):1146-54.

4 Schorah C. Commentary: from controversy and procrastination to primary prevention. Int J Epidemiol. 2011 Oct;40(5):1156-8. ("Schorah 2011").

5 Schorah 2011.

6 Czeizel AE, Dudás I. Prevention of the first occurrence of neural-tube defects by periconceptional vitamin supplementation. N Engl J Med. 1992 Dec 24;327(26):1832-5; de Bree A, van Dusseldorp M, Brouwer IA, van het Hof KH, Steegers-Theunissen RP. Folate intake in Europe: recommended, actual and desired intake. Eur J Clin Nutr. 1997 Oct;51(10):643-60.

7 http://www.cdc.gov/ncbddd/folicacid/recommendations.html http://www.nhs.uk/Conditions/vitamins-minerals/Pages/Vitamin-B.aspx

8 Ebisch IM, Thomas CM, Peters WH, Braat DD, Steegers-Theunissen RP. The importance of folate, zinc and antioxidants in the pathogenesis and prevention of subfertility. Hum Reprod Update. 2007 Mar-Apr;13(2):163-74 ("Ebisch 2007").

9 Chavarro JE, Rich-Edwards JW, Rosner BA, Willett WC. Use of multivitamins, intake of B vitamins, and risk of ovulatory infertility. Fertil Steril. 2008 Mar;89(3):668-76.

10  Westphal LM, Polan ML, Trant AS, Mooney SB. A nutritional supplement for improving fertility in women: a pilot study. J Reprod Med. 2004 Apr;49(4):289-93.
    Czeizel AE, Métneki J, Dudás I. The effect of preconceptional multivitamin supplementation on fertility. Int J Vitam Nutr Res. 1996;66(1):55-8.

11  Gaskins AJ, Mumford SL, Chavarro JE, Zhang C, Pollack AZ, Wactawski-Wende J, Perkins NJ, Schisterman EF. The impact of dietary folate intake on reproductive function in premenopausal women: a prospective cohort study. PLoS One. 2012;7(9):e46276. ("Gaskins 2012").

12  Gaskins 2012.

13  Ebisch 2007.

14  Boxmeer JC, Brouns RM, Lindemans J, Steegers EA, Martini E, Macklon NS, Steegers-Theunissen RP. Preconception folic acid treatment affects the microenvironment of the maturing oocyte in humans. Fertil Steril. 2008 Jun;89(6):1766-70. ("Boxmeer 2008").

15  Enciso M, Sarasa J, Xanthopoulou L, Bristow S, Bowles M, Fragouli E, Delhanty J, Wells D. Polymorphisms in the MTHFR gene influence embryo viability and the incidence of aneuploidy. Human genetics. 2016 May 1;135(5):555-68.

16  Yang, Y., Luo, Y., Yuan, J., Tang, Y., Xiong, L., Xu, M.,...& Liu, H. (2016). Association between maternal, fetal and paternal MTHFR gene C677T and A1298C polymorphisms and risk of recurrent pregnancy loss: a comprehensive evaluation. Archives of gynecology and obstetrics, 293(6), 1197-1211.
    Puri, M., Kaur, L., Walia, G. K., Mukhopadhhyay, R., Sachdeva, M. P., Trivedi, S. S.,...& Saraswathy, K. N. (2013). MTHFR C677T polymorphism, folate, vitamin B12 and homocysteine in recurrent pregnancy losses: a case control study among North Indian women. Journal of perinatal medicine, 41(5), 549-554.
    Al-Achkar, W., Wafa, A., Ammar, S., Moassass, F., & Jarjour, R. A. (2017). Association of methylenetetrahydrofolate reductase C677T and A1298C gene polymorphisms with recurrent pregnancy loss in Syrian women. Reproductive Sciences, 24(9), 1275-1279.
    Luo, L., Chen, Y., Wang, L., Zhuo, G., Qiu, C., Tu, Q.,...& Wang, X. (2015). Polymorphisms of genes involved in the folate metabolic pathway impact the occurrence of unexplained recurrent pregnancy loss. Reproductive Sciences, 22(7), 845-851.
    Chen, H., Yang, X., & Lu, M. (2016). Methylenetetrahydrofolate reductase gene polymorphisms and recurrent pregnancy loss

in China: a systematic review and meta-analysis. Archives of gynecology and obstetrics, 293(2), 283-290.

Cao, Y., Xu, J., Zhang, Z., Huang, X., Zhang, A., Wang, J.,... & Du, J. (2013). Association study between methylenetetrahydrofolate reductase polymorphisms and unexplained recurrent pregnancy loss: a meta-analysis. Gene, 514(2), 105-111.

Unfried, G., Griesmacher, A., Weismüller, W., Nagele, F., Huber, J. C., & Tempfer, C. B. (2002). The C677T polymorphism of the methylenetetrahydrofolate reductase gene and idiopathic recurrent miscarriage. Obstetrics & Gynecology, 99(4), 614-619.

17 Dell'Edera, D., L'Episcopia, A., Simone, F., Lupo, M. G., Epifania, A. A., & Allegretti, A. (2018). Methylenetetrahydrofolate reductase gene C677T and A1298C polymorphisms and susceptibility to recurrent pregnancy loss. Biomedical reports, 8(2), 172-175.

18 Zetterberg, H. (2004). Methylenetetrahydrofolate reductase and transcobalamin genetic polymorphisms in human spontaneous abortion: biological and clinical implications. Reproductive Biology and Endocrinology, 2(1), 7.

Govindaiah, V., Naushad, S. M., Prabhakara, K., Krishna, P. C., & Devi, A. R. R. (2009). Association of parental hyperhomocysteinemia and C677T Methylene tetrahydrofolate reductase (MTHFR) polymorphism with recurrent pregnancy loss. Clinical biochemistry, 42(4-5), 380-386.

Dell'Edera, D., L'Episcopia, A., Simone, F., Lupo, M. G., Epifania, A. A., & Allegretti, A. (2018). Methylenetetrahydrofolate reductase gene C677T and A1298C polymorphisms and susceptibility to recurrent pregnancy loss. Biomedical reports, 8(2), 172-175.

19 Dell'Edera, D., Tinelli, A., Milazzo, G. N., Malvasi, A., Domenico, C., Pacella, E.,... & Epifania, A. A. (2013). Effect of multivitamins on plasma homocysteine in patients with the 5, 10 methylenetetrahydrofolate reductase C677T homozygous state. Molecular medicine reports, 8(2), 609-612.

20 Mtiraoui, N., Zammiti, W., Ghazouani, L., Braham, N. J., Saidi, S., Finan, R. R.,... & Mahjoub, T. (2006). Methylenetetrahydrofolate reductase C677T and A1298C polymorphism and changes in homocysteine concentrations in women with idiopathic recurrent pregnancy losses. Reproduction, 131(2), 395-401.

Yang, Y., Luo, Y., Yuan, J., Tang, Y., Xiong, L., Xu, M.,... & Liu, H. (2016). Association between maternal, fetal and paternal MTHFR gene C677T and A1298C polymorphisms and risk of recurrent pregnancy loss: a comprehensive evaluation. Archives of gynecology and obstetrics, 293(6), 1197-1211.

Hwang, K. R., Choi, Y. M., Kim, J. J., Lee, S. K., Yang, K. M.,
Paik, E. C.,...& Hong, M. A. (2017). Methylenetetrahydrofolate
reductase polymorphisms and risk of recurrent pregnancy loss:
a case-control study. Journal of Korean medical science, 32(12),
2029-2034.
Al-Achkar, W., Wafa, A., Ammar, S., Moassass, F., & Jarjour, R. A.
(2017). Association of methylenetetrahydrofolate reductase C677T
and A1298C gene polymorphisms with recurrent pregnancy loss in
Syrian women. Reproductive Sciences, 24(9), 1275-1279.
Puri, M., Kaur, L., Walia, G. K., Mukhopadhhyay, R., Sachdeva,
M. P., Trivedi, S. S.,...& Saraswathy, K. N. (2013). MTHFR C677T
polymorphism, folate, vitamin B12 and homocysteine in recurrent
pregnancy losses: a case control study among North Indian
women. Journal of perinatal medicine, 41(5), 549-554.
21 Smith, D., Hornstra, J., Rocha, M., Jansen, G., Assaraf, Y., Lasry,
I.,...& Smulders, Y. M. (2017). Folic Acid Impairs the Uptake of
5-Methyltetrahydrofolate in Human Umbilical Vascular Endothelial
Cells. Journal of cardiovascular pharmacology, 70(4), 271.
22 Hekmatdoost A, Vahid F, Yari Z, Sadeghi M, Eini-Zinab H,
Lakpour N, Arefi S. Methyltetrahydrofolate vs Folic Acid
Supplementation in Idiopathic Recurrent Miscarriage with Respect
to Methylenetetrahydrofolate Reductase C677T and A1298C
Polymorphisms: A Randomized Controlled Trial. PloS one. 2015
Dec 2;10(12):e0143569.
23 Kos, B. J., Leemaqz, S. Y., McCormack, C. D., Andraweera, P.
H., Furness, D. L., Roberts, C. T., & Dekker, G. A. (2018). The
association of parental methylenetetrahydrofolate reductase
polymorphisms (MTHFR 677C> T and 1298A> C) and fetal loss:
a case–control study in South Australia. The Journal of Maternal-
Fetal & Neonatal Medicine, 1-6.
24 Puri, M., Kaur, L., Walia, G. K., Mukhopadhhyay, R., Sachdeva,
M. P., Trivedi, S. S.,...& Saraswathy, K. N. (2013). MTHFR C677T
polymorphism, folate, vitamin B12 and homocysteine in recurrent
pregnancy losses: a case control study among North Indian
women. Journal of perinatal medicine, 41(5), 549-554.
25 Patanwala, I., King, M. J., Barrett, D. A., Rose, J., Jackson,
R., Hudson, M.,...& Jones, D. E. (2014). Folic acid handling
by the human gut: implications for food fortification and
supplementation–. The American journal of clinical nutrition,
100(2), 593-599.
26 Smith, D., Hornstra, J., Rocha, M., Jansen, G., Assaraf, Y., Lasry,
I.,...& Smulders, Y. M. (2017). Folic Acid Impairs the Uptake of

5-Methyltetrahydrofolate in Human Umbilical Vascular Endothelial Cells. Journal of cardiovascular pharmacology, 70(4), 271.

27 Patanwala, I., King, M. J., Barrett, D. A., Rose, J., Jackson, R., Hudson, M.,...& Jones, D. E. (2014). Folic acid handling by the human gut: implications for food fortification and supplementation–. The American journal of clinical nutrition, 100(2), 593-599.

28 Boxmeer JC, Macklon NS, Lindemans J, Beckers NG, Eijkemans MJ, Laven JS, Steegers EA, Steegers-Theunissen RP. IVF outcomes are associated with biomarkers of the homocysteine pathway in monofollicular fluid. Hum Reprod. 2009 May;24(5):1059-66.

## Chapter 6: Energize Your Eggs with Coenzyme Q10

1 Dietmar A, Schmidt ME, Siebrecht SC. Ubiquinol supplementation enhances peak power production in trained athletes: a double-blind, placebo controlled study. J Int Soc Sports Nutr. 2013 Apr 29;10(1):24.

2 Bentinger M, Brismar K, Dallner G. The antioxidant role of coenzyme Q. Mitochondrion. 2007 Jun;7 Suppl:S41-50; Sohal RS. Coenzyme Q and vitamin E interactions. Methods Enzymol. 2004;378:146-51.

3 Shigenaga MK, Hagen TM, Ames BN.Oxidative damage and mitochondrial decay in aging.Proc Natl Acad Sci U S A. 1994 Nov 8;91(23):10771 8.
Seo AY, Joseph AM, Dutta D, Hwang JC, Aris JP, Leeuwenburgh C.New insights into the role of mitochondria in aging: mitochondrial dynamics and more.J Cell Sci. 2010 Aug 1;123(Pt 15):2533-42 ("Seo 2010").

4 Seo 2010

5 Tatone C, Amicarelli F, Carbone MC, Monteleone P, Caserta D, Marci R, Artini PG, Piomboni P, Focarelli R. Cellular and molecular aspects of ovarian follicle ageing. Hum Reprod Update. 2008 Mar-Apr;14(2):131-42.

6 Wilding M, Dale B, Marino M, di Matteo L, Alviggi C, Pisaturo ML, Lombardi L, De Placido G. Mitochondrial aggregation patterns and activity in human oocytes and preimplantation embryos. Hum Reprod. 2001 May;16(5):909-17 ("Wilding 2001").

7 de Bruin JP, Dorland M, Spek ER, Posthuma G, van Haaften M, Looman CW, te Velde ER. Age-related changes in the ultrastructure of the resting follicle pool in human ovaries. Biol Reprod. 2004 Feb;70(2):419-24 ("deBruin 2004").

8 Wilding 2001.

9   Bentov Y, Casper RF.The aging oocyte—can mitochondrial function be improved? Fertil Steril. 2013 Jan;99(1):18-22. ("Bentov 2013").

10  Bonomi M, Somigliana E, Cacciatore C, Busnelli M, Rossetti R, Bonetti S, Paffoni A, Mari D, Ragni G, Persani L; Italian Network for the study of Ovarian Dysfunctions. Blood cell mitochondrial DNA content and premature ovarian aging. PLoS One. 2012;7(8):e42423

11  Van Blerkom J, Davis PW, Lee J. ATP content of human oocytes and developmental potential and outcome after in-vitro fertilization and embryo transfer. Hum Reprod. 1995 Feb;10(2):415-24

12  Santos TA, El Shourbagy A, St John JC. Mitochondrial content reflects oocyte variability and fertilization outcome. Fertil Steril. 2006;85:584–91; Bentov Y, Esfandiari N, Burstein E, Casper RF.The use of mitochondrial nutrients to improve the outcome of infertility treatment in older patients.fertil Steril. 2010 Jan;93(1):272-5 ("Bentov 2010").

13  Dumollard R, Carroll J, Duchen MR, Campbell K, Swann K. Mitochondrial function and redox state in mammalian embryos. Semin Cell Dev Biol. 2009 May;20(3):346-53.

14  Van Blerkom J. Mitochondrial function in the human oocyte and embryo and their role in developmental competence. Mitochondrion. 2011 Sep;11(5):797-813 ("Van Blerkom 2011").

15  Eichenlaub-Ritter U, Vogt E, Yin H, Gosden R. Spindles, mitochondria and redox potential in ageing oocytes. Reprod Biomed Online. 2004 Jan;8(1):45-58; Van Blerkom 2011; Ge H, Tollner TL, Hu Z, Dai M, Li X, Guan H, Shan D, Zhang X, Lv J, Huang C, Dong Q. The importance of mitochondrial metabolic activity and mitochondrial DNA replication during oocyte maturation in vitro on oocyte quality and subsequent embryo developmental competence. Mol Reprod Dev. 2012 Jun;79(6):392-401.

16  Wilding M, Placido G, Matteo L, Marino M, Alviggi C, Dale B. Chaotic mosaicism in human preimplantation embryos is correlated with a low mitochondrial membrane potential. Fertil Steril. 2003;79:340–6 ("Wilding 2003").
    Zeng HT, Ren Z, Yeung WS, Shu YM, Xu YW, Zhuang GL, Liang XY. Low mitochondrial DNA and ATP contents contribute to the absence of birefringent spindle imaged with PolScope in in vitro matured human oocytes. Hum Reprod. 2007 Jun;22(6):1681-6.

17  Yu Y, Dumollard R, Rossbach A, Lai FA, Swann K. Redistribution of mitochondria leads to bursts of ATP production during

spontaneous mouse oocyte maturation. J Cell Physiol. 2010 Sep;224(3):672-80.

18 Wilding 2003.

19 Zhang X, Wu XQ, Lu S, Guo YL, Ma X. Deficit of mitochondria-derived ATP during oxidative stress impairs mouse MII oocyte spindles. Cell Res. 2006 Oct;16(10):841-50.

20 Eichenlaub-Ritter U, Vogt E, Yin H, Gosden R. Spindles, mitochondria and redox potential in ageing oocytes. Reprod Biomed Online. 2004 Jan;8(1):45-58.

21 Bartmann AK, Romao GS, Ramos Eda S, Ferriani RA. Why do older women have poor implantation rates? A possible role of the mitochondria. J Assist Reprod Genet. 2004;21:79–83; Thundathil J, Filion F, Smith LC.Molecular control of mitochondrial function in preimplantation mouse embryos.Mol Reprod Dev. 2005 Aug;71(4):405-13.

22 Thouas GA, Trounson AO, Wolvetang EJ, Jones GM. Mitochondrial dysfunction in mouse oocytes results in preimplantation embryo arrest in vitro. Biol Reprod. 2004 Dec;71(6):1936-42; Eichenlaub-Ritter U, Wieczorek M, Lüke S, Seidel T. Age related changes in mitochondrial function and new approaches to study redox regulation in mammalian oocytes in response to age or maturation conditions. Mitochondrion. 2011 Sep;11(5):783-96.

23 Interview with Dr. Bentov, published May 16, 2011, http://www.chatelaine.com/health/what-every-woman-over-30-should-know-about-fertility/

24 Bentov 2010; Bentov 2013.

25 Quinzii CM, Hirano M, DiMauro S. CoQ10 deficiency diseases in adults. Mitochondrion. 2007;7(Suppl):S122–6; Lopez 2010, Bergamini 2012, Shigenaga MK, Hagen TM, Ames BN. Oxidative damage and mitochondrial decay in aging. Proc Natl Acad Sci U S A. 1994 Nov 8;91(23):10771-8.

26 Perez-Sanchez C, Ruiz-Limon P, Aguirre MA, Bertolaccini ML, Khamashta MA, Rodriguez-Ariza A, Segui P, Collantes-Estevez E, Barbarroja N, Khraiwesh H, Gonzalez-Reyes JA, Villalba JM, Velasco F, Cuadrado MJ, Lopez-Pedrera C. Mitochondrial dysfunction in antiphospholipid syndrome: implications in the pathogenesis of the disease and effects of coenzyme Q(10) treatment. Blood. 2012 Jun 14;119(24):5859-70.

27 Akarsu, S., Gode, F., Isik, A. Z., Dikmen, Z. G., & Tekindal, M. A. (2017). The association between coenzyme Q10 concentrations in follicular fluid with embryo morphokinetics and pregnancy rate in

assisted reproductive techniques. Journal of assisted reproduction and genetics, 34(5), 599-605.

Turi A, Giannubilo SR, Brugè F, Principi F, Battistoni S, Santoni F, Tranquilli AL, Littarru G, Tiano L.Coenzyme Q10 content in follicular fluid and its relationship with oocyte fertilization and embryo grading.Arch Gynecol Obstet. 2012 Apr;285(4):1173-6

28  Bentov 2010, Bentov 2013.

29  Xu, Y., Nisenblat, V., Lu, C., Li, R., Qiao, J., Zhen, X., & Wang, S. (2018). Pretreatment with coenzyme Q10 improves ovarian response and embryo quality in low-prognosis young women with decreased ovarian reserve: a randomized controlled trial. Reproductive Biology and Endocrinology, 16(1), 29

Giannubilo, S., Orlando, P., Silvestri, S., Cirilli, I., Marcheggiani, F., Ciavattini, A., & Tiano, L. (2018). CoQ10 Supplementation in Patients Undergoing IVF-ET: The Relationship with Follicular Fluid Content and Oocyte Maturity. Antioxidants, 7(10), 141

30  Bentov, Y., Hannam, T., Jurisicova, A., Esfandiari, N., & Casper, R. F. (2014). Coenzyme Q10 supplementation and oocyte aneuploidy in women undergoing IVF-ICSI treatment. Clinical Medicine Insights: Reproductive Health, 8, CMRH-S14681.

31  McGarry, A., McDermott, M., Kieburtz, K., de Blieck, E. A., Beal, F., Marder, K.,...& Guttman, M. (2017). A randomized, double-blind, placebo-controlled trial of coenzyme Q10 in Huntington disease. Neurology, 88(2), 152-159.

Yeung, C. K., Billings, F. T., Claessens, A. J., Roshanravan, B., Linke, L., Sundell, M. B.,...& Himmelfarb, J. (2015). Coenzyme Q 10 dose-escalation study in hemodialysis patients: safety, tolerability, and effect on oxidative stress. BMC nephrology, 16(1), 183.

Seet, R. C. S., Lim, E. C., Tan, J. J., Quek, A. M., Chow, A. W., Chong, W. L.,...& Halliwell, B. (2014). Does high-dose coenzyme Q10 improve oxidative damage and clinical outcomes in Parkinson's disease?.

32  Aberg F, Appelkvist EL, Dallner G, Ernster L. Distribution and redox state of ubiquinones in rat and human tissues. Arch Biochem Biophys. 1992 Jun;295(2):230-4; Miles MV, Horn PS, Morrison JA, Tang PH, DeGrauw T, Pesce AJ. Plasma coenzyme Q10 reference intervals, but not redox status, are affected by gender and race in self-reported healthy adults. Clin Chim Acta. 2003 Jun;332(1-2):123-32.

33  Zhang, Y., Liu, J., Chen, X. Q., & Chen, C. Y. O. (2018). Ubiquinol is superior to ubiquinone to enhance Coenzyme Q10 status in older men. Food & function.

Langsjoen, P. H., & Langsjoen, A. M. (2014). Comparison study of plasma coenzyme Q10 levels in healthy subjects supplemented with ubiquinol versus ubiquinone. Clinical pharmacology in drug development, 3(1), 13-17

34 Villalba JM, Parrado C, Santos-Gonzalez M, Alcain FJ. Therapeutic use of coenzyme Q10 and coenzyme Q10-related compounds and formulations. Expert Opin Investig Drugs. 2010 Apr;19(4):535-54.

35 Bergamini C, Moruzzi N, Sblendido A, Lenaz G, Fato R. A water soluble CoQ10 formulation improves intracellular distribution and promotes mitochondrial respiration in cultured cells. PLoS One. 2012;7(3):e33712; Chopra RK, Goldman R, Sinatra ST, Bhagavan HN. Relative bioavailability of coenzyme Q10 formulations in human subjects. Int J Vitam Nutr Res. 1998;68(2):109-13., Bhagavan 2006;

36 López-Lluch, G., del Pozo-Cruz, J., Sánchez-Cuesta, A., Cortés-Rodríguez, A. B., & Navas, P. (2019). Bioavailability of coenzyme Q10 supplements depends on carrier lipids and solubilization. Nutrition, 57, 133-140.

37 Singh, R. B., Niaz, M. A., Kumar, A., Sindberg, C. D., Moesgaard, S., & Littarru, G. P. (2005). Effect on absorption and oxidative stress of different oral Coenzyme Q10 dosages and intake strategy in healthy men. Biofactors, 25(1-4), 219-224.

38 Spindler M, Beal MF, Henchcliffe C. Coenzyme Q10 effects in neurodegenerative disease. Neuropsychiatr Dis Treat. 2009;5:597-610 ("Spindler 2009"); Hosoe 2007.

39 Ferrante KL, Shefner J, Zhang H, Betensky R, O'Brien M, Yu H, Fantasia M, Taft J, Beal MF, Traynor B, Newhall K, Donofrio P, Caress J, Ashburn C, Freiberg B, O'Neill C, Paladenech C, Walker T, Pestronk A, Abrams B, Florence J, Renna R, Schierbecker J, Malkus B, Cudkowicz M. Tolerance of high-dose (3,000 mg/day) coenzyme Q10 in ALS. Neurology. 2005 Dec 13;65(11):1834-6, Spindler 2009.

40 Reinhold, C. M. (2018). Coenzyme Q10 Supplementation in Orthostatic Hypotension and Multiple-System Atrophy: A Report on 7 Cases. The American journal of medicine, 131(4), 444-446.

41 Mezawa M, Takemoto M, Onishi S, Ishibashi R, Ishikawa T, Yamaga M, Fujimoto M, Okabe E, He P, Kobayashi K, Yokote K. The reduced form of coenzyme Q10 improves glycemic control in patients with type 2 diabetes: an open label pilot study. Biofactors. 2012 Nov-Dec;38(6):416-21.

42 Molyneux SL, Young JM, Florkowski CM, Lever M, George PM. Coenzyme Q10: is there a clinical role and a case for measurement? Clin Biochem Rev. 2008 May;29(2):71-82.

43  Pérez-Sánchez, C., Aguirre, M. Á., Ruiz-Limón, P., Ábalos-Aguilera, M. C., Jiménez-Gómez, Y., Arias-de la Rosa, I., ... & Collantes-Estévez, E. (2017). Ubiquinol effects on antiphospholipid syndrome prothrombotic profile: a randomized, placebo-controlled trial. Arteriosclerosis, thrombosis, and vascular biology, ATVBAHA-117

## Chapter 7: Melatonin and Other Antioxidants

1   Evans H. The pioneer history of vitamin E. Vitam Horm. 1963;20:379–387.
2   de Bruin JP, Dorland M, Spek ER, Posthuma G, van Haaften M, Looman CW, te Velde ER. Age-related changes in the ultrastructure of the resting follicle pool in human ovaries. Biol Reprod. 2004 Feb;70(2):419-24. ("de Bruin 2004").
3   Tatone C, Carbone MC, Falone S, Aimola P, Giardinelli A, Caserta D, Marci R, Pandolfi A, Ragnelli AM, Amicarelli F. Age-dependent changes in the expression of superoxide dismutases and catalase are associated with ultrastructural modifications in human granulosa cells. Mol Hum Reprod. 2006 Nov;12(11):655-60. Carbone MC, Tatone C, Delle Monache S, Marci R, Caserta D, Colonna R, Amicarelli F. Antioxidant enzymatic defences in human follicular fluid: characterization and age-dependent changes. Mol Hum Reprod. 2003 Nov;9(11):639-43.
4   Shigenaga MK, Hagen TM, Ames BN.Oxidative damage and mitochondrial decay in aging. Proc Natl Acad Sci U S A. 1994 Nov 8;91(23):10771-8.
5   Agarwal A, Aponte-Mellado A, Premkumar BJ, Shaman A, Gupta S. The effects of oxidative stress on female reproduction: a review. Reprod Biol Endocrinol. 2012 Jun 29;10:49. ("Agarwal 2012.")
6   Bentov Y, Casper RF.The aging oocyte—can mitochondrial function be improved? Fertil Steril. 2013 Jan;99(1):18-22. ("Bentov 2013").
7   Polak G, Koziol-Montewka M, Gogacz M, Blaszkowska I, Kotarski J. Total antioxidant status of peritoneal fluid in infertile women. Eur J Obstet Gynecol Reprod Biol. 2001;94:261–263. Wang Y, Sharma RK, Falcone T, Goldberg J, Agarwal A. Importance of reactive oxygen species in the peritoneal fluid of women with endometriosis or idiopathic infertility. Fertil Steril. 1997;68:826–830. ("Wang 1997"). Paszkowski T, Traub AI, Robinson SY, McMaster D. Selenium dependent glutathione peroxidase activity in human follicular fluid. Clin Chim Acta. 1995;236(2):173–180. doi: 10.1016/0009-8981(95)98130-9. ("Paszkowski 1995").

8   Kumar K, Deka D, Singh A, Mitra DK, Vanitha BR, Dada
    R.Predictive value of DNA integrity analysis in idiopathic
    recurrent pregnancy loss following spontaneous conception. J
    Assist Reprod Genet. 2012 Sep;29(9):861-7.
9   Zhang X, Wu XQ, Lu S, Guo YL, Ma X.Deficit of mitochondria-
    derived ATP during oxidative stress impairs mouse MII oocyte
    spindles.Cell Res. 2006 Oct;16(10):841-50.
10  Agarwal 2012; Wang 1997.
11  Augoulea A, Mastorakos G, Lambrinoudaki I, Christodoulakos G,
    Creatsas G. The role of the oxidative-stress in the endometriosis-
    related infertility. Gynecol Endocrinol. 2009;25:75 -81.); Bedaiwy
    MA, Falcone T. Peritoneal fluid environment in endometriosis.
    clinicopathological implications. Minerva Ginecol. 2003;55:333-45.
    Rajani S, Chattopadhyay R, Goswami SK, Ghosh S, Sharma S,
    Chakravarty B. Assessment of oocyte quality in polycystic ovarian
    syndrome and endometriosis by spindle imaging and reactive
    oxygen species levels in follicular fluid and its relationship with
    IVF-ET outcome. J Hum Reprod Sci. 2012 May;5(2):187-93.
    ("Rajani 2012").
    Wang Y, Sharma RK, Falcone T, Goldberg J, Agarwal A.
    Importance of reactive oxygen species in the peritoneal fluid of
    women with endometriosis or idiopathic infertility. Fertil Steril.
    1997;68:826–30.
    Van Langendonckt A, Casanas-Roux F, Donnez J. Oxidative stress
    and peritoneal endometriosis. Fertil Steril. 2002;77:861–70.
12  González-Comadran, M., Schwarze, J. E., Zegers-Hochschild, F.,
    Maria do Carmo, B. S., Carreras, R., & Checa, M. Á. (2017). The
    impact of endometriosis on the outcome of Assisted Reproductive
    Technology. Reproductive Biology and Endocrinology, 15(1), 8.
    Senapati, S., Sammel, M. D., Morse, C., & Barnhart, K. T. (2016).
    Impact of endometriosis on in vitro fertilization outcomes: an
    evaluation of the Society for Assisted Reproductive Technologies
    Database. Fertility and sterility, 106(1), 164-171.
13  Xu, B., Guo, N., Zhang, X. M., Shi, W., Tong, X. H., Iqbal, F.,
    & Liu, Y. S. (2015). Oocyte quality is decreased in women with
    minimal or mild endometriosis. Scientific reports, 5, 10779.
    Sanchez, A. M., Vanni, V. S., Bartiromo, L., Papaleo, E., Zilberberg,
    E., Candiani, M.,... & Viganò, P. (2017). Is the oocyte quality
    affected by endometriosis? A review of the literature. Journal of
    ovarian research, 10(1), 43.
14  Song, Y., Liu, J., Qiu, Z., Chen, D., Luo, C., Liu, X.,... & Liu, W.
    (2018). Advanced oxidation protein products from the follicular

microenvironment and their role in infertile women with
endometriosis. Experimental and therapeutic medicine, 15(1), 479-486.
Da Broi, M. G., Jordão-Jr, A. A., Ferriani, R. A., & Navarro,
P. A. (2018). Oocyte oxidative DNA damage may be involved
in minimal/mild endometriosis–related infertility. Molecular
reproduction and development, 85(2), 128-136.

15  Victor VM, Rocha M, Banuls C, Alvarez A, de Pablo C, Sanchez-
Serrano M, Gomez M, Hernandez-Mijares A. Induction of
oxidative stress and human leukocyte/endothelial cell interactions
in polycystic ovary syndrome patients with insulin resistance. J
Clin Endocrinol Metab. 2011;96:3115–3122. ("Victor 2011").

16  Gonzalez F, Rote NS, Minium J, Kirwan JP. Reactive oxygen
species-induced oxidative stress in the development of insulin
resistance and hyperandrogenism in polycystic ovary syndrome. J
Clin Endocrinol Metab. 2006;91:336–340.
Palacio JR, Iborra A, Ulcova-Gallova Z, Badia R, Martinez P. The
presence of antibodies to oxidative modified proteins in serum
from polycystic ovary syndrome patients. Clin Exp Immunol.
2006;144:217–222.

17  Victor 2011., Rajani 2012.

18  Patel SM, Nestler JE. Fertility in polycystic ovary syndrome.
Endocrinol Metab Clin North Am. 2006;35:137–55.
Wood JR, Dumesic DA, Abbott DH, Strauss JF., III Molecular
abnormalities in oocytes from women with polycystic ovary
syndrome revealed by microarray analysis. J Clin Endocrinol
Metab. 2007;92:705–13.

19  Wiener-Megnazi Z, Vardi L, Lissak A, Shnizer S, Reznick
AZ, Ishai D, Lahav-Baratz S, Shiloh H, Koifman M, Dirnfeld
M. Oxidative stress indices in follicular fluid as measured by
the thermochemiluminescence assay correlate with outcome
parameters in in vitro fertilization. Fertil Steril. 2004;82(Suppl
3):1171–1176.
de Bruin 2004, Eichenlaub 2011, premkumar 2012, Carbone 2003,
Tatone 2006,

20  Wang LY, Wang DH, Zou XY, Xu CM. Mitochondrial functions on
oocytes and preimplantation embryos. J Zhejiang Univ Sci B. 2009
Jul;10(7):483-92.

21  Shaum KM, Polotsky AJ.Nutrition and reproduction: is there
evidence to support a "Fertility Diet" to improve mitochondrial
function? Maturitas. 2013 Apr;74(4):309-12.

22  E.g.: Ruder EH, Hartman TJ, Reindollar RH, Goldman MB.
Female dietary antioxidant intake and time to pregnancy among

couples treated for unexplained infertility. Fertil Steril. 2013 Dec 17 [Epub ahead of print]. ("Ruder 2014").

23 Aydin Y, Ozatik O, Hassa H, Ulusoy D, Ogut S, Sahin F.Relationship between oxidative stress and clinical pregnancy in assisted reproductive technology treatment cycles. J Assist Reprod Genet. 2013 Jun;30(6):765-72.

24 Ruder 2014.

25 Chemineau P, Guillaume D, Migaud M, Thiéry JC, Pellicer-Rubio MT, Malpaux B. Seasonality of reproduction in mammals: intimate regulatory mechanisms and practical implications. Reprod Domest Anim. 2008 Jul;43 Suppl 2:40-7.

26 Brzezinski A, Seibel MM, Lynch HJ, Deng MH, Wurtman RJ. Melatonin in human preovulatory follicular fluid. J Clin Endocrinol Metab. 1987;64(4):865–867.
Ronnberg L, Kauppila A, Leppaluoto J, Martikainen H, Vakkuri O. Circadian and seasonal variation in human preovulatory follicular fluid melatonin concentration. J Clin Endocrinol Metab. 1990;71(2):492–496.

27 Nakamura Y, Tamura H, Takayama H, Kato H. Increased endogenous level of melatonin in preovulatory human follicles does not directly influence progesterone production. Fertil Steril. 2003 Oct;80(4):1012-6.

28 Tamura H, Takasaki A, Taketani T, Tanabe M, Kizuka F, Lee L, Tamura I, Maekawa R, Aasada H, Yamagata Y, Sugino N. The role of melatonin as an antioxidant in the follicle. J Ovarian Res. 2012 Jan 26;5:5. ("Tamura 2012").

29 Poeggeler B, Reiter RJ, Tan DX, Chen LD, Manchester LC. Melatonin, hydroxyl radical-mediated oxidative damage, and aging: a hypothesis. J Pineal Res. 1993;14(4):151–168.
Schindler AE, Christensen B, Henkel A, Oettel M, Moore C. High-dose pilot study with the novel progestogen dienogestin patients with endometriosis. Gynecol Endocrinol. 2006;22(1):9–17.

30 Reiter RJ, Tan DX, Manchester LC, Qi W. Biochemical reactivity of melatonin with reactive oxygen and nitrogen species: a review of the evidence. Cell Biochem Biophys. 2001;34(2):237–256.
Tan DX, Manchester LC, Reiter RJ, Plummer BF, Limson J, Weintraub ST, Qi W. Melatonin directly scavenges hydrogen peroxide: a potentially new metabolic pathway of melatonin biotransformation. Free Radic Biol Med. 2000;29(11):1177–1185. ("Tan 2000").

31 Tan 2000.

32  Sack RL, Lewy AJ, Erb DL, Vollmer WM, Singer CM. Human melatonin production decreases with age. J Pineal Res. 1986;3(4):379-88.

33  Tong, J., Sun, Y., Li, H., Li, W. P., Zhang, C., & Chen, Z. (2017). Melatonin levels in follicular fluid as markers for IVF outcomes and predicting ovarian reserve. Reproduction, REP-16.

34  Tamura H, Takasaki A, Miwa I, Taniguchi K, Maekawa R, Asada H, Taketani T, Matsuoka A, Yamagata Y, Shimamura K. et al. Oxidative stress impairs oocyte quality and melatonin protects oocytes from free radical damage and improves fertilization rate. J Pineal Res. 2008;44(3):280-287 ("Tamura 2008")
Jahnke G, Marr M, Myers C, Wilson R, Travlos G, Price C. Maternal and developmental toxicity evaluation of melatonin administered orally to pregnant Sprague-Dawley rats. Toxicol Sci. 1999;50(2):271-279.
Ishizuka B, Kuribayashi Y, Murai K, Amemiya A, Itoh MT. The effect of melatonin on in vitro fertilization and embryo development in mice. J Pineal Res. 2000;28(1):48-51
Papis K, Poleszczuk O, Wenta-Muchalska E, Modlinski JA. Melatonin effect on bovine embryo development in vitro in relation to oxygen concentration. J Pineal Res. 2007;43(4):321-326.
Shi JM, Tian XZ, Zhou GB, Wang L, Gao C, Zhu SE, Zeng SM, Tian JH, Liu GS. Melatonin exists in porcine follicular fluid and improves in vitro maturation and parthenogenetic development of porcine oocytes. J Pineal Res. 2009;47(4):318-323.

35  Tamura 2012.

36  Tamura 2008; Tamura 2012.

37  Tamura 2012.

38  Interview with Dr. Tamura, published on September 15, 2010, http://www.news-medical.net/news/20100915/Hormone-melatonin-improves-egg-quality-in-IVF.aspx

39  Rizzo P, Raffone E, Benedetto V.Effect of the treatment with myo-inositol plus folic acid plus melatonin in comparison with a treatment with myo-inositol plus folic acid on oocyte quality and pregnancy outcome in IVF cycles. A prospective, clinical trial.Eur Rev Med Pharmacol Sci. 2010 Jun;14(6):555-61.
Nishihara, T., Hashimoto, S., Ito, K., Nakaoka, Y., Matsumoto, K., Hosoi, Y., & Morimoto, Y. (2014). Oral melatonin supplementation improves oocyte and embryo quality in women undergoing in vitro fertilization-embryo transfer. Gynecological endocrinology, 30(5), 359-362.

Jahromi, B. N., Sadeghi, S., Alipour, S., Parsanezhad, M. E., & Alamdarloo, S. M. (2017). Effect of melatonin on the outcome of assisted reproductive technique cycles in women with diminished ovarian reserve: A double-blinded randomized clinical trial. Iranian journal of medical sciences, 42(1), 73.

Fernando, S., Wallace, E. M., Vollenhoven, B., Lolatgis, N., Hope, N., Wong, M.,... & Thomas, P. (2018). Melatonin in Assisted Reproductive Technology: A Pilot Double-Blind Randomized Placebo-Controlled Clinical Trial. Frontiers in endocrinology, 9.

Eryilmaz, O. G., Devran, A., Sarikaya, E., Aksakal, F. N., Mollamahmutoğlu, L., & Cicek, N. (2011). Melatonin improves the oocyte and the embryo in IVF patients with sleep disturbances, but does not improve the sleeping problems. Journal of assisted reproduction and genetics, 28(9), 815.

Batıoğlu, A. S., Şahin, U., Gürlek, B., Öztürk, N., & Ünsal, E. (2012). The efficacy of melatonin administration on oocyte quality. Gynecological Endocrinology, 28(2), 91-93.

40  Schwertner, A., Dos Santos, C. C. C., Costa, G. D., Deitos, A., de Souza, A., de Souza, I. C. C.,... & Caumo, W. (2013). Efficacy of melatonin in the treatment of endometriosis: a phase II, randomized, double-blind, placebo-controlled trial. PAIN®, 154(6), 874-881.

41  Cetinkaya, N., Attar, R., Yildirim, G., Ficicioglu, C., Ozkan, F., Yilmaz, B., & Yesildaglar, N. (2015). The effects of different doses of melatonin treatment on endometrial implants in an oophorectomized rat endometriosis model. Archives of gynecology and obstetrics, 291(3), 591-598.

Yilmaz, B., Kilic, S., Aksakal, O., Ertas, I. E., Tanrisever, G. G., Aksoy, Y.,... & Gungor, T. (2015). Melatonin causes regression of endometriotic implants in rats by modulating angiogenesis, tissue levels of antioxidants and matrix metalloproteinases. Archives of gynecology and obstetrics, 292(1), 209-216

Yesildaglar, N., Yıldırım, G., Yildirim, O. K., Attar, R., Ozkan, F., Akkaya, H., & Yilmaz, B. (2016). The effects of melatonin on endometriotic lesions induced by implanting human endometriotic cells in the first SCID-mouse endometriosis-model developed in Turkey. Clinical and experimental obstetrics & gynecology, 43(1), 25-30.

42  Woo MM, Tai CJ, Kang SK, Nathwani PS, Pang SF, Leung PC.Direct action of melatonin in human granulosa-luteal cells.J Clin Endocrinol Metab. 2001 Oct;86(10):4789-97.

43  Tagliaferri, V., Romualdi, D., Scarinci, E., Cicco, S. D., Florio, C. D., Immediata, V.,... & Apa, R. (2018). Melatonin treatment may

be able to restore menstrual cyclicity in women with PCOS: a pilot study. Reproductive Sciences, 25(2), 269-275..

44  Pacchiarotti, A., Carlomagno, G., Antonini, G., & Pacchiarotti, A. (2016). Effect of myo-inositol and melatonin versus myo-inositol, in a randomized controlled trial, for improving in vitro fertilization of patients with polycystic ovarian syndrome. Gynecological endocrinology, 32(1), 69-73.

45  Nishihara, T., Hashimoto, S., Ito, K., Nakaoka, Y., Matsumoto, K., Hosoi, Y., & Morimoto, Y. (2014). Oral melatonin supplementation improves oocyte and embryo quality in women undergoing in vitro fertilization-embryo transfer. Gynecological endocrinology, 30(5), 359-362.

46  Jahromi, B. N., Sadeghi, S., Alipour, S., Parsanezhad, M. E., & Alamdarloo, S. M. (2017). Effect of melatonin on the outcome of assisted reproductive technique cycles in women with diminished ovarian reserve: A double-blinded randomized clinical trial. Iranian journal of medical sciences, 42(1), 73.

47  Natarajan 2010; Olson SE, Seidel GE., Jr Culture of in vitro-produced bovine embryos with vitamin E improves development in vitro and after transfer to recipients. Biol Reprod. 2000;62(2):248–252.

48  Tamura H, Takasaki A, Miwa I, Taniguchi K, Maekawa R, Asada H, Taketani T, Matsuoka A, Yamagata Y, Shimamura K, Morioka H, Ishikawa H, Reiter RJ, Sugino N. Oxidative stress impairs oocyte quality and melatonin protects oocytes from free radical damage and improves fertilization rate. J Pineal Res. 2008 Apr;44(3):280-7.

49  http://www.efsa.europa.eu/en/efsajournal/pub/640.htm

50  Mayo Clinic, 2012, Vitamin E Dosing. Available at http://www.mayoclinic.com/health/vitamin-e/NS_patient-vitamine/DSECTION=dosing

51  Colorado Center for Reproductive Medicine. Female Fertility Supplements. 2012. http://www.colocrm.com/FertilitySupplements.aspx

52  Ruder EH, Hartman TJ, Reindollar RH, Goldman MB. Female dietary antioxidant intake and time to pregnancy among couples treated for unexplained infertility. Fertil Steril. 2013 Dec 17 [Epub ahead of print]. ("Ruder 2014").

53  Yeh J, Bowman MJ, Browne RW, Chen N. Reproductive aging results in a reconfigured ovarian antioxidant defense profile in rats. Fertil Steril. 2005 Oct;84 Suppl 2:1109-13; Ruder 2014.

54  Luck MR, Jeyaseelan I, Scholes RA. Ascorbic acid and fertility. Biol Reprod. 1995 Feb;52(2):262-6; Zreik TG, Kodaman PH, Jones EE, Olive DL, Behrman H. Identification and characterization of an ascorbic acid transporter in human granulosa-lutein cells. Mol Hum Reprod. 1999 Apr;5(4):299-302.

55  Tarín J, Ten J, Vendrell FJ, de Oliveira MN, Cano A. Effects of maternal ageing and dietary antioxidant supplementation on ovulation, fertilisation and embryo development in vitro in the mouse. Reprod Nutr Dev. 1998 Sep-Oct;38(5):499-508; Tarín JJ, Pérez-Albalá S, Cano A. Oral antioxidants counteract the negative effects of female aging on oocyte quantity and quality in the mouse. Mol Reprod Dev. 2002 Mar;61(3):385-97; Ozkaya MO, Nazıroğlu M. Multivitamin and mineral supplementation modulates oxidative stress and antioxidant vitamin levels in serum and follicular fluid of women undergoing in vitro fertilization. Fertil Steril. 2010 Nov;94(6):2465-6.

56  Ruder 2014.

57  Lu, X., Wu, Z., Wang, M., & Cheng, W. (2018). Effects of vitamin C on the outcome of in vitro fertilization–embryo transfer in endometriosis: A randomized controlled study. Journal of International Medical Research, 46(11), 4624-4633.

58  Bentov Y, Esfandiari N, Burstein E, Casper RF.The use of mitochondrial nutrients to improve the outcome of infertility treatment in older patients. Fertil Steril. 2010 Jan;93(1):272-5 ("Bentov 2010.")

59  Goraca A, Huk-Kolega H, Piechota A, Kleniewska P, Ciejka E, et al. (2011) Lipoic acid - biological activity and therapeutic potential. Pharmacol Rep 63: 849–858.

60  Packer L, Witt EH, Tritschler HJ: -Lipoic acid as a biological antioxidant. Free Radic Biol Med, 1995, 19, 227–250.

61  Arivazhagan P, Ramanathan K, Panneerselvam C: Effect of DL—lipoic acid on mitochondrial enzymes in aged rats. Chem Biol Interact, 2001, 138, 189–198. Mc Carthy MF, Barroso-Aranda J, Contreras F: The "rejuvenatory" impact of lipoic acid on mitochondrial function in aging rats may reflect induction and activation of PPAR-coactivator-1. Med Hypotheses, 2009, 72, 29–33

62  Zembron-Lacny A, Slowinska-Lisowska M, Szygula Z, Witkowski K, Szyszka K. The comparison of antioxidant and hematological properties of N-acetylcysteine and alpha-lipoic acid in physically

active males. Physiol Res Academ Sci Bohemoslov. 2009;58(6):855–861; Sun 2012. Zhang 2013

63  Talebi A, Zavareh S, Kashani MH, Lashgarbluki T, Karimi I.The effect of alpha lipoic acid on the developmental competence of mouse isolated preantral follicles. J Assist Reprod Genet. 2012 Feb;29(2):175-83.
Zhang H, Wu B, Liu H, Qiu M, Liu J, Zhang Y, Quan F. Improving development of cloned goat embryos by supplementing α-lipoic acid to oocyte in vitro maturation medium. Theriogenology. 2013 Aug;80(3):228-33.

64  Haghighian, H. K., Haidari, F., Mohammadi-asl, J., & Dadfar, M. (2015). Randomized, triple-blind, placebo-controlled clinical trial examining the effects of alpha-lipoic acid supplement on the spermatogram and seminal oxidative stress in infertile men. Fertility and sterility, 104(2), 318-324.

65  Rago, R., Marcucci, I., Leto, G., Caponecchia, L., Salacone, P., Bonanni, P.,...& Sebastianelli, A. (2015). Effect of myo-inositol and alpha-lipoic acid on oocyte quality in polycystic ovary syndrome non-obese women undergoing in vitro fertilization: a pilot study. J Biol Regul Homeost Agents, 29(4), 913-923.

66  De Cicco, S., Immediata, V., Romualdi, D., Policola, C., Tropea, A., Di Florio, C.,...& Apa, R. (2017). Myoinositol combined with alpha-lipoic acid may improve the clinical and endocrine features of polycystic ovary syndrome through an insulin-independent action. Gynecological Endocrinology, 33(9), 698-701.

67  Masharani U, Gjerde C, Evans JL, Youngren JF, Goldfine ID. Effects of controlled-release alpha lipoic acid in lean, nondiabetic patients with polycystic ovary syndrome. J Diabetes Sci Technol. 2010 Mar 1;4(2):359-64.

68  Pınar, N., Soylu Karapınar, O., Özcan, O., Özgür, T., & Bayraktar, S. (2017). Effect of alpha–lipoic acid on endometrial implants in an experimental rat model. Fundamental & clinical pharmacology, 31(5), 506-512.
Lete, I., Mendoza, N., de la Viuda, E., & Carmona, F. (2018). Effectiveness of an antioxidant preparation with N-acetyl cysteine, alpha lipoic acid and bromelain in the treatment of endometriosis-associated pelvic pain: LEAP study. European Journal of Obstetrics & Gynecology and Reproductive Biology, 228, 221-224.

69  Ghibu S, Richard C, Vergely C, Zeller M, Cottin Y, Rochette L: Antioxidant properties of an endogenous thiol: Alpha-lipoic acid, useful in the prevention of cardiovascular diseases. J Cardiovasc Pharmacol, 2009, 54, 391–398.

Shay KP, Moreau RF, Smith EJ, Smith AR, Hagen TM: Alpha-lipoic acid as a dietary supplement: Molecular mechanisms and therapeutic potential. Biochim Biophys Acta, 2009, 1790, 1149–1160.
Ziegler D, Nowak H, Kempler P, Vargha P & Low PA. Treatment of symptomatic diabetic polyneuropathy with the antioxidant α-lipoic acid: a meta-analysis. Diabetic Medicine 2004 21 114–121.

70  Segermann J, Hotze A, Ulrich H, et al. Effect of alpha-lipoic acid on the peripheral conversion of thyroxine to triiodothyronine and on serum lipid-, protein- and glucose levels. Arzneimittelforschung. 1991;41:1294-1298.

71  Porasuphatana S, Suddee S, Nartnampong A, et al. Gylcemic and oxidative status of patients with type 2 diabetes mellitus following oral administration of alpha-lipoic acid: a randomized double-blinded placebo-controlled study. *Asia Pac J Clin Nutr* 2012;21(1):12–21.
Golbidi S, Badran M, Laher I. Diabetes and alpha lipoic Acid. Front Pharmacol. 2011;2:69.

72  Goraca A, Huk-Kolega H, Piechota A, Kleniewska P, Ciejka E, et al. (2011) Lipoic acid - biological activity and therapeutic potential. Pharmacol Rep 63: 849–858.

73  Gleiter CH, Schug BS, Hermann R, Elze M, Blume HH, Gundert-Remy U: Influence of food intake on the bioa- vailability of thioctic acid enantiomers (letter). Eur J Clin Pharmacol, 1996, 50, 513-514

74  Atkuri KR, Mantovani JJ, Herzenberg LA, Herzenberg LA.N-Acetylcysteine—a safe antidote for cysteine/glutathione deficiency. Curr Opin Pharmacol. 2007 Aug;7(4):355-9. ("Atkuri 2007").

75  Dodd S, Dean O, Copolov DL, Malhi GS, Berk M.N-acetylcysteine for antioxidant therapy: pharmacology and clinical utility. Expert Opin Biol Ther. 2008 Dec;8(12):1955-62.
Atkuri 2007.

76  Thakker, D., Raval, A., Patel, I., & Walia, R. (2015). N-acetylcysteine for polycystic ovary syndrome: a systematic review and meta-analysis of randomized controlled clinical trials. Obstetrics and gynecology international, 2015.
Mostajeran, F., Tehrani, H. G., & Rahbary, B. (2018). N-Acetylcysteine as an Adjuvant to Letrozole for Induction of Ovulation in Infertile Patients with Polycystic Ovary Syndrome. Advanced biomedical research, 7.
Cheraghi, E., Mehranjani, M. S., Shariatzadeh, M. A., Esfahani, M. H. N., & Ebrahimi, Z. (2016). N-Acetylcysteine improves oocyte and embryo quality in polycystic ovary syndrome patients undergoing

intracytoplasmic sperm injection: an alternative to metformin. Reproduction, Fertility and Development, 28(6), 723-731 Nasr A. Effect of N-acetyl-cysteine after ovarian drilling in clomiphene citrate-resistant PCOS women: a pilot study.Reprod Biomed Online. 2010 Mar;20(3):403-9. ("Nasr 2010").

77  Salehpour S, Sene AA, Saharkhiz N, Sohrabi MR, Moghimian F.N-Acetylcysteine as an adjuvant to clomiphene citrate for successful induction of ovulation in infertile patients with polycystic ovary syndrome.J Obstet Gynaecol Res. 2012 Sep;38(9):1182-6.

78  Hebisha, S. A., Omran, M. S., Sallam, H. N., & Ahmed, A. I. (2015). Follicular fluid homocysteine levels with N-Acetyl cysteine supplemented controlled ovarian hyperstimulation, correlation with oocyte yield and ICSI cycle outcome. Fertility and Sterility, 104(3), e324.:

79  Amin AF, Shaaban OM, Bediawy MA.N-acetyl cysteine for treatment of recurrent unexplained pregnancy loss. Reprod Biomed Online. 2008 Nov;17(5):722-6.

80  Nasr 2010.

81  Giorgi, V. S., Da Broi, M. G., Paz, C. C., Ferriani, R. A., & Navarro, P. A. (2016). N-acetyl-cysteine and L-carnitine prevent meiotic oocyte damage induced by follicular fluid from infertile women with mild endometriosis. Reproductive Sciences, 23(3), 342-351.

82  Porpora, M. G., Brunelli, R., Costa, G., Imperiale, L., Krasnowska, E. K., Lundeberg, T.,... & Parasassi, T. (2013). A promise in the treatment of endometriosis: an observational cohort study on ovarian endometrioma reduction by N-acetylcysteine. Evidence-based Complementary and Alternative Medicine, 2013.

83  Dodd 2008, Atkuri 2007

84  Lynch RM, Robertson R. Anaphylactoid reactions to intravenous N-acetylcysteine: a prospective case controlled study.Accid Emerg Nurs. 2004 Jan;12(1):10-5.

85  Ismail, A. M., Hamed, A. H., Saso, S., & Thabet, H. H. (2014). Adding L-carnitine to clomiphene resistant PCOS women improves the quality of ovulation and the pregnancy rate. A randomized clinical trial. European Journal of Obstetrics & Gynecology and Reproductive Biology, 180, 148-152. Latifian, S., Hamdi, K., & Totakneh, R. (2015). Effect of addition of l-carnitine in polycystic ovary syndrome (PCOS) patients with clomiphene citrate and gonadotropin resistant. Int J Curr Res Acad Rev, 3, 469-76.

86 Fenkci, S. M., Fenkci, V., Oztekin, O., Rota, S., & Karagenc, N. (2008). Serum total L-carnitine levels in non-obese women with polycystic ovary syndrome. Human reproduction, 23(7), 1602-1606.
87 Agarwal, A., Sengupta, P., & Durairajanayagam, D. (2018). Role of L-carnitine in female infertility. Reproductive Biology and Endocrinology, 16(1), 5.
Dionyssopoulou, E., Vassiliadis, S., Evangeliou, A., Koumantakis, E. E., & Athanassakis, I. (2005). Constitutive or induced elevated levels of L-carnitine correlate with the cytokine and cellular profile of endometriosis. Journal of reproductive immunology, 65(2), 159-170.
Christiana, K., George, T., George, F., Margarita, T., Anna, T., Costas, F., & Irene, A. (2014). L-carnitine alters lipid body content in pre-implantation embryos leading to infertility. J Reprod Immunol, 101, 18-39.
88 Kitano, Y., Hashimoto, S., Matsumoto, H., Yamochi, T., Yamanaka, M., Nakaoka, Y.,... & Morimoto, Y. (2018). Oral administration of l-carnitine improves the clinical outcome of fertility in patients with IVF treatment. Gynecological Endocrinology, 1-5.
89 Lim J, Luderer U. Oxidative damage increases and antioxidant gene expression decreases with aging in the mouse ovary. Biol Reprod. 2011 Apr;84(4):775-82; Liu 2012.

## Chapter 8: Restoring Ovulation with Myo-Inositol

1 Mitchell Bebel Stargrove, Jonathan Treasure, Dwight L. McKee. Herb, Nutrient, and Drug Interactions: Clinical Implications and Therapeutic Strategies, Health Sciences, 2008, p. 765.
2 Chiu TT, Rogers MS, Law EL, Briton-Jones CM, Cheung LP, Haines CJ.Follicular fluid and serum concentrations of myo-inositol in patients undergoing IVF: relationship with oocyte quality.Hum Reprod. 2002 Jun;17(6):1591-6. ("Chiu 2002").
3 Lisi F, Carfagna P, Oliva MM, Rago R, Lisi R, Poverini R, Manna C, Vaquero E, Caserta D, Raparelli V, Marci R, Moscarini M.Pretreatment with myo-inositol in non polycystic ovary syndrome patients undergoing multiple follicular stimulation for IVF: a pilot study. Reprod Biol Endocrinol. 2012 Jul 23;10:52. ("Lisi 2012").
Caprio, F., D'Eufemia, M. D., Trotta, C., Campitiello, M. R., Ianniello, R., Mele, D., & Colacurci, N. (2015). Myo-inositol therapy for poor-responders during IVF: a prospective controlled observational trial. Journal of ovarian research, 8(1), 37
4 Caprio, F., D'Eufemia, M. D., Trotta, C., Campitiello, M. R., Ianniello, R., Mele, D., & Colacurci, N. (2015). Myo-inositol

therapy for poor-responders during IVF: a prospective controlled observational trial. Journal of ovarian research, 8(1), 37

5   Papaleo E, Unfer V, Baillargeon JP, Fusi F, Occhi F, De Santis L.Myo-inositol may improve oocyte quality in intracytoplasmic sperm injection cycles. A prospective, controlled, randomized trial. Fertil Steril. 2009 May;91(5):1750-4; ("Papaleo 2009").
    Genazzani AD, Lanzoni C, Ricchieri F, Jasonni VM. Myo-inositol administration positively affects hyperinsulinemia and hormonal parameters in overweight patients with polycystic ovary syndrome. Gynecol Endocrinol. 2008 Mar;24(3):139-44. ("Genazzani 2008").

6   Baptiste CG, Battista MC, Trottier A, Baillargeon JP. Insulin and hyperandrogenism in women with polycystic ovary syndrome. J Steroid Biochem Mol Biol. 2010 Oct;122(1-3):42-52.
    Filicori M, Flamigni C, Campaniello E, Meriggiola MC, Michelacci L, Valdiserri A, Ferrari P. Polycystic ovary syndrome: abnormalities and management with pulsatile gonadotropin-releasing hormone and gonadotropin-releasing hormone analogs. Am J Obstet Gynecol. 1990 Nov;163(5 Pt 2):1737-42.

7   Hasegawa I, Murakawa H, Suzuki M, Yamamoto Y, Kurabayashi T, Tanaka K. Effect of troglitazone on endocrine and ovulatory performance in women with insulin resistance-related polycystic ovary syndrome. Fertil Steril. 1999 Feb;71(2):323-7.
    Ng EH, Wat NM, Ho PC. Effects of metformin on ovulation rate, hormonal and metabolic profiles in women with clomiphene-resistant polycystic ovaries: a randomized, double-blinded placebo-controlled trial. Hum Reprod. 2001 Aug;16(8):1625-31.
    Lord JM, Flight IH, Norman RJ. Metformin in polycystic ovary syndrome: systematic review and meta-analysis. BMJ. 2003 Oct 25;327(7421):951-3.

8   Fleming R, Hopkinson ZE, Wallace AM, Greer IA, Sattar N. Ovarian function and metabolic factors in women with oligomenorrhea treated with metformin in a randomized double blind placebo-controlled trial. J Clin Endocrinol Metab 2002;87: 569-74.

9   Baillargeon JP, Diamanti-Kandarakis E, Ostlund RE Jr, Apridonidze T, Iuorno MJ, Nestler JE. Altered D-chiro-inositol urinary clearance in women with polycystic ovary syndrome. Diabetes Care. 2006 Feb;29(2):300-5; Constantino 2009.

10  Chiu TT, Rogers MS, Briton-Jones C, Haines C. Effects of myo-inositol on the in-vitro maturation and subsequent development of mouse oocytes. Hum Reprod. 2003 Feb;18(2):408-16.

11  Papaleo E, Unfer V, Baillargeon JP, De Santis L, Fusi F, Brigante C, Marelli G, Cino I, Redaelli A, Ferrari A. Myo-inositol in patients

with polycystic ovary syndrome: a novel method for ovulation induction. Gynecol Endocrinol. 2007 Dec;23(12):700-3.

12  Genazzani 2008.

13  Costantino D, Minozzi G, Minozzi E, Guaraldi C.Metabolic and hormonal effects of myo-inositol in women with polycystic ovary syndrome: a double-blind trial.Eur Rev Med Pharmacol Sci. 2009 Mar-Apr;13(2):105-10.

14  Papaleo 2009

15  Ciotta L, Stracquadanio M, Pagano I, Carbonaro A, Palumbo M, Gulino F.Effects of myo-inositol supplementation on oocyte's quality in PCOS patients: a double blind trial.Eur Rev Med Pharmacol Sci. 2011 May;15(5):509-14.

16  Unfer V, Carlomagno G, Rizzo P, Raffone E, Roseff S. Myo-inositol rather than D-chiro-inositol is able to improve oocyte quality in intracytoplasmic sperm injection cycles. A prospective, controlled, randomized trial. Eur Rev Med Pharmacol Sci. 2011 Apr;15(4):452-7.

17  D'Anna R, Di Benedetto V, Rizzo P, Raffone E, Interdonato ML, Corrado F, Di Benedetto A. Myo-inositol may prevent gestational diabetes in PCOS women. Gynecol Endocrinol. 2012 Jun;28(6):440-2

18  Craig LB, Ke RW, Kutteh WH.Increased prevalence of insulin resistance in women with a history of recurrent pregnancy loss. Fertil Steril. 2002 Sep;78(3):487-90. ("Craig 2002").

19  Craig 2002.

20  Liui 2012; Carlomagno G, Unfer V.Inositol safety: clinical evidences. Eur Rev Med Pharmacol Sci. 2011 Aug;15(8):931-6.

21  Isabella R, Raffone E. Does ovary need D-chiro-inositol? J Ovarian Res. 2012 May 15;5(1):14. ("Isabella 2012").

22  Galletta M, Grasso S, Vaiarelli A, Roseff SJ. Bye-bye chiro-inositol - myo-inositol: true progress in the treatment of polycystic ovary syndrome and ovulation induction. Eur Rev Med Pharmacol Sci. 2011 Oct;15(10):1212-4.

23  Isabella 2012

24  Kalra, B., Kalra, S., & Sharma, J. B. (2016). The inositols and polycystic ovary syndrome. Indian journal of endocrinology and metabolism, 20(5), 720.

25  Carlomagno G, Unfer V, Roseff S.The D-chiro-inositol paradox in the ovary.Fertil Steril. 2011 Jun 30;95(8):2515-6.

26  Nordio, M., & Proietti, E. (2012). The combined therapy with myo-inositol and D-chiro-inositol reduces the risk of metabolic disease in PCOS overweight patients compared to myo-inositol supplementation alone. Eur Rev Med Pharmacol Sci, 16(5), 575-81.

## Chapter 9: DHEA for Diminished Ovarian Reserve

1   Fouany MR, Sharara FI. Is there a role for DHEA supplementation in women with diminished ovarian reserve? J Assist Reprod Genet. 2013 Sep;30(9):1239-44.

2   http://www.centerforhumanreprod.com/dhea.html

3   Harper AJ, Buster JE, Casson PR. Changes in adrenocortical function with aging and therapeutic implications. Semin Reprod Endocrinol. 1999;17(4):327-38.

4   Gleicher, N., Kushnir, V. A., Weghofer, A., & Barad, D. H. (2016). The importance of adrenal hypoandrogenism in infertile women with low functional ovarian reserve: a case study of associated adrenal insufficiency. Reproductive Biology and Endocrinology, 14(1), 23.

5   Casson PR, Lindsay MS, Pisarska MD, Carson SA, Buster JE. Dehydroepiandrosterone supplementation augments ovarian stimulation in poor responders: a case series. Hum Reprod 2000;15:2129-2132.

6   Barad DH, et al, Update on the use of dehydroepiandrosterone supplementation among women with diminished ovarian reserve. J Assist Reprod Genet 2007;24(12):629-34.

7   http://www.centerforhumanreprod.com/dhea.html, interview with CBS News.

8   http://www.centerforhumanreprod.com/dhea.html, interview with CBS News.

9   Gleicher N, Barad DH. Dehydroepiandrosterone (DHEA) supplementation in diminished ovarian reserve (DOR). Reprod Biol Endocrinol. 2011 May 17;9:67 ("Gleicher 2011").

10  Gleicher 2011

11  Barad DH and Gleicher N, Effects of dehydroepiandrosterone on oocyte and embryo yields, embryo grade and cell number in IVF. Hum Reprod 2006;21(11):2845-9.

12  Barad DH, et al, Update on the use of dehydroepiandrosterone supplementation among women with diminished ovarian reserve. J Assist Reprod Genet 2007;24(12):629-34.

13  Zhang, M., Niu, W., Wang, Y., Xu, J., Bao, X., Wang, L.,...& Sun, Y. (2016). Dehydroepiandrosterone treatment in women with poor ovarian response undergoing IVF or ICSI: a systematic review and meta-analysis. Journal of assisted reproduction and genetics, 33(8), 981-991.

    Schwarze, J. E., Canales, J., Crosby, J., Ortega-Hrepich, C., Villa, S., & Pommer, R. (2018). DHEA use to improve likelihood of IVF/ICSI success in patients with diminished ovarian reserve: A systematic review and meta-analysis. JBRA assisted reproduction, 22(4), 369.

14  Kotb, M. M., Hassan, A. M., & AwadAllah, A. M. (2016). Does dehydroepiandrosterone improve pregnancy rate in women undergoing IVF/ICSI with expected poor ovarian response according to the Bologna criteria? A randomized controlled trial. European Journal of Obstetrics & Gynecology and Reproductive Biology, 200, 11-15.

15  Chern, C. U., Tsui, K. H., Vitale, S. G., Chen, S. N., Wang, P. H., Cianci, A.,... & Lin, L. T. (2018). Dehydroepiandrosterone (DHEA) supplementation improves in vitro fertilization outcomes of poor ovarian responders, especially in women with low serum concentration of DHEA-S: a retrospective cohort study. Reproductive Biology and Endocrinology, 16(1), 90.

16  Zhang, M., Niu, W., Wang, Y., Xu, J., Bao, X., Wang, L.,... & Sun, Y. (2016). Dehydroepiandrosterone treatment in women with poor ovarian response undergoing IVF or ICSI: a systematic review and meta-analysis. Journal of assisted reproduction and genetics, 33(8), 981-991.
Schwarze, J. E., Canales, J., Crosby, J., Ortega-Hrepich, C., Villa, S., & Pommer, R. (2018). DHEA use to improve likelihood of IVF/ICSI success in patients with diminished ovarian reserve: A systematic review and meta-analysis. JBRA assisted reproduction, 22(4), 369.

17  Bedaiwy MA, Ryan E, Shaaban O, Claessens EA, Blanco-Mejia S, Casper RF: Follicular conditioning with dehydroepiandrosterone co-treatment improves IUI outcome in clomiphene citrate patients. 55th Annual Meeting of the Canadian Fertility and Andrology Society, Montreal, Canada, November 18-21, 2009.

18  Fusi FM, Ferrario M, Bosisio C, Arnoldi M, Zanga L. DHEA supplementation positively affects spontaneous pregnancies in women with diminished ovarian function. Gynecol Endocrinol. 2013 Oct;29(10):940-3 ("Fusi 2013").

19  Barad 2007.

20  Barad 2007; Fusi 2013.

21  Gleicher N, et al, Miscarriage rates after dehydroepiandrosterone (DHEA) supplementation in women with diminished ovarian reserve: a case control study. Reprod Biol Endocrinol 2009;7(7):108 ("Gleicher 2009").

22  Levi AJ, Raynault MF, Bergh PA, Drews MR, Miller BT, Scott RT Jr: Reproductive outcome in patients with diminished ovarian reserve. Fertil Steril 2001, 76:666-669.

23 Gleicher N, et al, Dehydroepiandrosterone (DHEA) reduces embryo aneuploidy: direct evidence from preimplantation genetic screening (PGS). Reprod Biol Endocrinol 2010;10(8):140 ("Gleicher 2010a")
Gleicher 2009.

24 Gleicher 2010a.

25 Gleicher 2010a.

26 Zhang, M., Niu, W., Wang, Y., Xu, J., Bao, X., Wang, L.,...& Sun, Y. (2016). Dehydroepiandrosterone treatment in women with poor ovarian response undergoing IVF or ICSI: a systematic review and meta-analysis. Journal of assisted reproduction and genetics, 33(8), 981-991.
Schwarze, J. E., Canales, J., Crosby, J., Ortega-Hrepich, C., Villa, S., & Pommer, R. (2018). DHEA use to improve likelihood of IVF/ICSI success in patients with diminished ovarian reserve: A systematic review and meta-analysis. JBRA assisted reproduction, 22(4), 369.

27 Sen A, Hammes SR: Granulosa cell-specific androgen receptors are critical regulators of development and function. Mol Endocrinol 2010, 24:1393-1403.

28 Hyman 2013.

29 Gleicher 2011.

30 Grunwald, K., Feldmann, K., Melsheimer, P., Rabe, T., Neulen, J., & Runnebaum, B. (1998). Aneuploidy in human granulosa lutein cells obtained from gonadotrophin-stimulated follicles and its relation to intrafollicular hormone concentrations. Human reproduction (Oxford, England), 13(10), 2679-2687.

31 Wald NJ. Commentary: a brief history of folic acid in the prevention of neural tube defects. Int J Epidemiol. 2011 Oct;40(5):1154-6;
Schorah C. Commentary: from controversy and procrastination to primary prevention. Int J Epidemiol. 2011 Oct;40(5):1156-8.

32 Gleicher 2010a.

33 Yilmaz N, Uygur D, Inal H, Gorkem U, Cicek N, Mollamahmutoglu L. Dehydroepiandrosterone supplementation improves predictive markers for diminished ovarian reserve: serum AMH, inhibin B and antral follicle count. Eur J Obstet Gynecol Reprod Biol. 2013 Jul;169(2):257-60; Fouany 2013.

34 Gleicher 2011.

35 Yakin 2011.

36 Gleicher 2011

37 Gleicher 2011.

38  Wiser 2010.
39  Panjari M, Bell RJ, Jane F, Adams J, Morrow C, Davis SR: The safety of 52 weeks of oral DHEA therapy for postmenopausal women. Maturitas 2009, 63:240-245.
40  Franasiak, J. M., Thomas, S., Ng, S., Fano, M., Ruiz, A., Scott, R. T., & Forman, E. J. (2016). Dehydroepiandrosterone (DHEA) supplementation results in supraphysiologic DHEA-S serum levels and progesterone assay interference that may impact clinical management in IVF. Journal of assisted reproduction and genetics, 33(3), 387-391.
41  Rao, K. A. (2018). DHEA supplementation in a woman with endometriosis desiring pregnancy. MEDICINE, 25(9), 24.
42  https://www.centerforhumanreprod.com/fertility/endometriosis-infertility-monthly-case-report/
43  Gleicher, N., Kushnir, V. A., Darmon, S. K., Wang, Q., Zhang, L., Albertini, D. F., & Barad, D. H. (2017). New PCOS-like phenotype in older infertile women of likely autoimmune adrenal etiology with high AMH but low androgens. The Journal of steroid biochemistry and molecular biology, 167, 144-152.
44  Parasrampuria J, Schwartz K, Petesch R. Quality control of dehydroepiandrosterone dietary supplement products. JAMA. 1998 Nov 11;280(18):1565.
45  Casson PR, Straughn AB, Umstot ES, Abraham GE, Carson SA, Buster JE. Delivery of dehydroepiandrosterone to premenopausal women: effects of micronization and nonoral administration. Am J Obstet Gynecol. 1996 Feb;174(2):649-53.
46  Gleicher 2011; Wiser 2010.

## Chapter 10: Supplements That May Do More Harm Than Good

1  http://www.pycnogenol.com/science/research-library/
2  Blank S, Bantleon FI, McIntyre M, Ollert M, Spillner E. The major royal jelly proteins 8 and 9 (Api m 11) are glycosylated components of Apis mellifera venom with allergenic potential beyond carbohydrate-based reactivity. Clin Exp Allergy. 2012 Jun;42(6):976-85.
3  Morita H, Ikeda T, Kajita K, Fujioka K, Mori I, Okada H, Uno Y, Ishizuka T. Effect of royal jelly ingestion for six months on healthy volunteers. Nutr J. 2012 Sep 21;11:77.
4  Battaglia C, Salvatori M, Maxia N, Petraglia F, Facchinetti F, Volpe A. Adjuvant

L-arginine treatment for in-vitro fertilization in poor responder patients. Hum Reprod. 1999 Jul;14(7):1690-7. ("Battaglia 1999").

5  Battaglia 1999.

6  Keay, S.D., Liversedge, N.H., Mathur, R.S. and Jenkins, J.M. Assisted conception following poor ovarian response to gonadotrophin stimulation. Br. J. Obstet. Gynecol. 1997,104, 521–527; Tanbo T, Abyholm T, Bjøro T, Dale PO. Ovarian stimulation in previous failures from in-vitro fertilization: distinction of two groups of poor responders. Hum Reprod. 1990 Oct;5(7):811-5.

7  Battaglia 1999.

8  Battaglia C, Regnani G, Marsella T, Facchinetti F, Volpe A, Venturoli S, Flamigni C. Adjuvant L-arginine treatment in controlled ovarian hyperstimulation: a double-blind, randomized study.Hum Reprod. 2002 Mar;17(3):659-65.

9  Agarwal A, Gupta S, Sekhon L, Shah R. Redox considerations in female reproductive function and assisted reproduction: from molecular mechanisms to health implications. Antioxid Redox Signal. 2008 Aug;10(8):1375-403.

10  Bódis J, Várnagy A, Sulyok E, Kovács GL, Martens-Lobenhoffer J, Bode-Böger SM.Negative association of L-arginine methylation products with oocyte numbers.Hum Reprod. 2010 Dec;25(12):3095-100. doi: 10.1093/humrep/deq257. Epub 2010 Sep 24.

11  Lee TH, Wu MY, Chen MJ, Chao KH, Ho HN, Yang YS. Nitric oxide is associated with poor embryo quality and pregnancy outcome in in vitro fertilization cycles. Fertil Steril. 2004 Jul;82(1):126-31.

## Chapter 11: Preparing for Embryo Transfer

1  Shapiro, B. S., Daneshmand, S. T., Garner, F. C., Aguirre, M., Hudson, C., & Thomas, S. (2011). Evidence of impaired endometrial receptivity after ovarian stimulation for in vitro fertilization: a prospective randomized trial comparing fresh and frozen–thawed embryo transfer in normal responders. Fertility and sterility, 96(2), 344-348.
Roque, M., Lattes, K., Serra, S., Solà, I., Geber, S., Carreras, R., & Checa, M. A. (2013). Fresh embryo transfer versus frozen embryo transfer in in vitro fertilization cycles: a systematic review and meta-analysis. Fertility and sterility, 99(1), 156-162.

2  Coates, A., Kung, A., Mounts, E., Hesla, J., Bankowski, B., Barbieri, E.,... & Munné, S. (2017). Optimal euploid embryo transfer strategy, fresh versus frozen, after preimplantation

genetic screening with next generation sequencing: a randomized controlled trial. Fertility and sterility, 107(3), 723-730.

Roque, M., Valle, M., Guimarães, F., Sampaio, M., & Geber, S. (2015). Freeze-all policy: fresh vs. frozen-thawed embryo transfer. Fertility and sterility, 103(5), 1190-1193.

Wang, A., Santistevan, A., Cohn, K. H., Copperman, A., Nulsen, J., Miller, B. T.,... & Beim, P. Y. (2017). Freeze-only versus fresh embryo transfer in a multicenter matched cohort study: contribution of progesterone and maternal age to success rates. Fertility and sterility, 108(2), 254-261

3 Wang, A., Santistevan, A., Cohn, K. H., Copperman, A., Nulsen, J., Miller, B. T.,... & Beim, P. Y. (2017). Freeze-only versus fresh embryo transfer in a multicenter matched cohort study: contribution of progesterone and maternal age to success rates. Fertility and sterility, 108(2), 254-261.

4 Bu, Z., Wang, K., Dai, W., & Sun, Y. (2016). Endometrial thickness significantly affects clinical pregnancy and live birth rates in frozen-thawed embryo transfer cycles. Gynecological Endocrinology, 32(7), 524-528.

5 Ribeiro, V. C., Santos-Ribeiro, S., De Munck, N., Drakopoulos, P., Polyzos, N. P., Schutyser, V.,... & Blockeel, C. (2018). Should we continue to measure endometrial thickness in modern-day medicine? The effect on live birth rates and birth weight. Reproductive biomedicine online, 36(4), 416-426.

6 Weiss, N. S., Van Vliet, M. N., Limpens, J., Hompes, P. G. A., Lambalk, C. B., Mochtar, M. H.,... & Van Wely, M. (2017). Endometrial thickness in women undergoing IUI with ovarian stimulation. How thick is too thin? A systematic review and meta-analysis. Human Reproduction, 32(5), 1009-1018.

7 Ma, N. Z., Chen, L., Dai, W., Bu, Z. Q., Hu, L. L., & Sun, Y. P. (2017). Influence of endometrial thickness on treatment outcomes following in vitro fertilization/intracytoplasmic sperm injection. Reproductive Biology and Endocrinology, 15(1), 5.

8 Hashemi, Z., Sharifi, N., Khani, B., Aghadavod, E., & Asemi, Z. (2019). The effects of vitamin E supplementation on endometrial thickness, and gene expression of vascular endothelial growth factor and inflammatory cytokines among women with implantation failure. The Journal of Maternal-Fetal & Neonatal Medicine, 32(1), 95-102.

9 Takasaki, A., Tamura, H., Miwa, I., Taketani, T., Shimamura, K., & Sugino, N. (2010). Endometrial growth and uterine blood flow:

a pilot study for improving endometrial thickness in the patients with a thin endometrium. Fertility and sterility, 93(6), 1851-1858.

10 El Refaeey, A., Selem, A., & Badawy, A. (2014). Combined coenzyme Q10 and clomiphene citrate for ovulation induction in clomiphene-citrate-resistant polycystic ovary syndrome. Reproductive biomedicine online, 29(1), 119-124.

11 Eid, M. E. (2015). Sildenafil improves implantation rate in women with a thin endometrium secondary to improvement of uterine blood flow;"pilot study". Fertility and Sterility, 104(3), e342. Mekled, A. K. H., Abd El-Rahim, A. M., & El-Sayed, A. (2017). Effect of Sildenafil Citrate on the Outcome of in vitro Fertilization after Multiple IVF Failures Attributed to Poor Endometrial Development: A Randomized Controlled Trial. Egyptian Journal of Hospital Medicine, 69(1).

12 Paulus, W. E., Zhang, M., Strehler, E., El-Danasouri, I., & Sterzik, K. (2002). Influence of acupuncture on the pregnancy rate in patients who undergo assisted reproduction therapy. Fertility and sterility, 77(4), 721-724.

13 Schwarze, J. E., Ceroni, J. P., Ortega-Hrepich, C., Villa, S., Crosby, J., & Pommer, R. (2018). Does acupuncture the day of embryo transfer affect the clinical pregnancy rate? Systematic review and meta-analysis. JBRA assisted reproduction, 22(4), 363. Manheimer, E., van der Windt, D., Cheng, K., Stafford, K., Liu, J., Tierney, J., ... & Bouter, L. M. (2013). The effects of acupuncture on rates of clinical pregnancy among women undergoing in vitro fertilization: a systematic review and meta-analysis. Human reproduction update, 19(6), 696-713. Shen, C., Wu, M., Shu, D., Zhao, X., & Gao, Y. (2015). The role of acupuncture in in vitro fertilization: a systematic review and meta-analysis. Gynecologic and obstetric investigation, 79(1), 1-12.

14 So, E. W. S., Ng, E. H. Y., Wong, Y. Y., Lau, E. Y. L., Yeung, W. S. B., & Ho, P. C. (2008). A randomized double blind comparison of real and placebo acupuncture in IVF treatment. Human Reproduction, 24(2), 341-348. So, E. W. S., Ng, E. H. Y., Wong, Y. Y., Yeung, W. S. B., & Ho, P. C. (2010). Acupuncture for frozen–thawed embryo transfer cycles: a double-blind randomized controlled trial. Reproductive biomedicine online, 20(6), 814-821.

15 Domar, A. D., Meshay, I., Kelliher, J., Alper, M., & Powers, R. D. (2009). The impact of acupuncture on in vitro fertilization outcome. Fertility and sterility, 91(3), 723-726.

16  Craig, L. B., Rubin, L. E., Peck, J. D., Anderson, M., Marshall, L. A., & Soules, M. R. (2014). Acupuncture performed before and after embryo transfer: a randomized controlled trial. The Journal of reproductive medicine, 59(5-6), 313-320.

17  Rubin, L. E. H., Anderson, B. J., & Craig, L. B. (2018). Acupuncture and in vitro fertilisation research: current and future directions. Acupuncture in Medicine, acupmed-2016.

Magarelli, P. C., Cridennda, D. K., & Cohen, M. (2009). Changes in serum cortisol and prolactin associated with acupuncture during controlled ovarian hyperstimulation in women undergoing in vitro fertilization–embryo transfer treatment. Fertility and Sterility, 92(6), 1870-1879.

di Villahermosa, D. I. M., dos Santos, L. G., Nogueira, M. B., Vilarino, F. L., & Barbosa, C. P. (2013). Influence of acupuncture on the outcomes of in vitro fertilisation when embryo implantation has failed: a prospective randomised controlled clinical trial. Acupuncture in Medicine, 31(2), 157-161.

18  Magarelli, P. C., Cridennda, D. K., & Cohen, M. (2009). Changes in serum cortisol and prolactin associated with acupuncture during controlled ovarian hyperstimulation in women undergoing in vitro fertilization–embryo transfer treatment. Fertility and Sterility, 92(6), 1870-1879.

## Chapter 13: The Egg Quality Diet

1  Hjollund NHI, Jensen TK, Bonde JPE, Henriksen NE, Andersson AM, Skakkebaek NE. Is glycosilated haemoglobin a marker of fertility? A follow-up study of first-pregnancy planners. Hum Reprod. 1999;14:1478–1482 ("Hjolland 1999").

2  Chavarro JE, Rich-Edwards JW, Rosner BA, Willett WC. A prospective study of dietary carbohydrate quantity and quality in relation to risk of ovulatory infertility. Eur J Clin Nutr. 2009 Jan;63(1):78-86 ("Chavarro 2009a").

3  Dumesic DA, Abbott DH. Implications of polycystic ovary syndrome on oocyte development. Semin Reprod Med. 2008 Jan;26(1):53-61.

4  Jinno 2011.

5  Jinno 2011.

6  Tatone C, Amicarelli F, Carbone MC, Monteleone P, Caserta D, Marci R, Artini PG, Piomboni P, Focarelli R. Cellular and molecular aspects of ovarian follicle ageing. Hum Reprod Update. 2008 Mar-Apr;14(2):131-42.

7   Wang Q, Moley KH. Maternal diabetes and oocyte quality. Mitochondrion. 2010 Aug;10(5):403-10 ("Wang 2010").

8   Craig LB, Ke RW, Kutteh WH. Increased prevalence of insulin resistance in women with a history of recurrent pregnancy loss. Fertil Steril. 2002 Sep;78(3):487-90.

9   Chakraborty P, Goswami SK, Rajani S, Sharma S, Kabir SN, Chakravarty B, Jana K. Recurrent pregnancy loss in polycystic ovary syndrome: role of hyperhomocysteinemia and insulin resistance. PLoS One. 2013 May 21;8(5):e64446; Tian L, Shen H, Lu Q, Norman RJ, Wang J. Insulin resistance increases the risk of spontaneous abortion after assisted reproduction technology treatment. J Clin Endocrinol Metab. 2007 Apr;92(4):1430-3.

10  Russell, J. B., Abboud, C., Williams, A., Gibbs, M., Pritchard, S., & Chalfant, D. (2012). Does changing a patient's dietary consumption of proteins and carbohydrates impact blastocyst development and clinical pregnancy rates from one cycle to the next?. Fertility and Sterility, 98(3), S47.

11  McGrice, M., & Porter, J. (2017). The effect of low carbohydrate diets on fertility hormones and outcomes in overweight and obese women: a systematic review. Nutrients, 9(3), 204.

12  Kose, E., Guzel, O., Demir, K., & Arslan, N. (2017). Changes of thyroid hormonal status in patients receiving ketogenic diet due to intractable epilepsy. Journal of Pediatric Endocrinology and Metabolism, 30(4), 411-416.

13  Machtinger, R., Gaskins, A. J., Mansur, A., Adir, M., Racowsky, C., Baccarelli, A. A., ... & Chavarro, J. E. (2017). Association between preconception maternal beverage intake and in vitro fertilization outcomes. Fertility and sterility, 108(6), 1026-1033.

14  Hatch, E. E., Wesselink, A. K., Hahn, K. A., Michiel, J. J., Mikkelsen, E. M., Sorensen, H. T., ... & Wise, L. A. (2018). Intake of Sugar-sweetened Beverages and Fecundability in a North American Preconception Cohort. Epidemiology, 29(3), 369-378.

15  Melanson KJ, Zukley L, Lowndes J, Nguyen V, Angelopoulos TJ, Rippe JM. Effects of high-fructose corn syrup and sucrose consumption on circulating glucose, insulin, leptin, and ghrelin and on appetite in normal-weight women. Nutrition. 2007;23:103–112. Stanhope KL, Griffen SC, Bair BR, Swarbrick MM, Keim NL, Havel PJ. Twenty-four-hour endocrine and metabolic profiles following consumption of high-fructose corn syrup-, sucrose-, fructose-, and glucose-sweetened beverages with meals. Am J Clin Nutr. 2008;87:1194–1203

16  Afeiche, M. C., Chiu, Y. H., Gaskins, A. J., Williams, P. L., Souter, I., Wright, D. L., ... & Chavarro, J. E. (2016). Dairy intake in relation to in vitro fertilization outcomes among women from a fertility clinic. Human Reproduction, 31(3), 563-571.

17  Estruch, R., Ros, E., Salas-Salvadó, J., Covas, M. I., Corella, D., Arós, F., ... & Lamuela-Raventos, R. M. (2013). Primary prevention of cardiovascular disease with a Mediterranean diet. New England Journal of Medicine, 368(14), 1279-1290.

Sofi, F., Abbate, R., Gensini, G. F., & Casini, A. (2010). Accruing evidence on benefits of adherence to the Mediterranean diet on health: an updated systematic review and meta-analysis. The American journal of clinical nutrition, 92(5), 1189-1196.

Schwingshackl, L., & Hoffmann, G. (2014). Adherence to Mediterranean diet and risk of cancer: A systematic review and meta–analysis of observational studies. International journal of cancer, 135(8), 1884-1897.

Tresserra-Rimbau, A., Rimm, E. B., Medina-Remón, A., Martínez-González, M. A., López-Sabater, M. C., Covas, M. I., ... & Arós, F. (2014). Polyphenol intake and mortality risk: a re-analysis of the PREDIMED trial. BMC medicine, 12(1), 77.

Martínez-González, M. Á., De la Fuente-Arrillaga, C., Nuñez-Cordoba, J. M., Basterra-Gortari, F. J., Beunza, J. J., Vazquez, Z., ... & Bes-Rastrollo, M. (2008). Adherence to Mediterranean diet and risk of developing diabetes: prospective cohort study. Bmj, 336(7657), 1348-1351.

18  Chrysohoou, C., Panagiotakos, D. B., Pitsavos, C., Das, U. N., & Stefanadis, C. (2004). Adherence to the Mediterranean diet attenuates inflammation and coagulation process in healthy adults: The ATTICA Study. Journal of the American College of Cardiology, 44(1), 152-158.

Richard, C., Couture, P., Desroches, S., & Lamarche, B. (2013). Effect of the Mediterranean diet with and without weight loss on markers of inflammation in men with metabolic syndrome. Obesity, 21(1), 51-57.

Sköldstam, L., Hagfors, L., & Johansson, G. (2003). An experimental study of a Mediterranean diet intervention for patients with rheumatoid arthritis. Annals of the rheumatic diseases, 62(3), 208-214.

19  Maxia, N., Uccella, S., Ersettigh, G., Fantuzzi, M., Manganini, M., Scozzesi, A., & Colognato, R. (2018). Can unexplained infertility be evaluated by a new immunological four-biomarkers panel? A pilot study. Minerva ginecologica, 70(2), 129-137.

Xie, J., Yan, L., Cheng, Z., Qiang, L., Yan, J., Liu, Y.,... & Hao, C. (2018). Potential effect of inflammation on the failure risk of in vitro fertilization and embryo transfer among infertile women. Human Fertility, 1-9.

Buyuk, E., Asemota, O. A., Merhi, Z., Charron, M. J., Berger, D. S., Zapantis, A., & Jindal, S. K. (2017). Serum and follicular fluid monocyte chemotactic protein-1 levels are elevated in obese women and are associated with poorer clinical pregnancy rate after in vitro fertilization: a pilot study. Fertility and sterility, 107(3), 632-640.

Wagner, M. M., Jukema, J. W., Hermes, W., le Cessie, S., de Groot, C. J., Bakker, J. A.,... & Bloemenkamp, K. W. (2018). Assessment of novel cardiovascular biomarkers in women with a history of recurrent miscarriage. Pregnancy hypertension, 11, 129-135.

See also: Ahmed, S. K., Mahmood, N., Malalla, Z. H., Alsobyani, F. M., Al-Kiyumi, I. S., & Almawi, W. Y. (2015). C-reactive protein gene variants associated with recurrent pregnancy loss independent of CRP serum levels: a case-control study. Gene, 569(1), 136-140.

Kushnir, V. A., Solouki, S., Sarig–Meth, T., Vega, M. G., Albertini, D. F., Darmon, S. K.,... & Gleicher, N. (2016). Systemic inflammation and autoimmunity in women with chronic endometritis. American Journal of Reproductive Immunology, 75(6), 672-677.

20 Karayiannis, D., Kontogianni, M. D., Mendorou, C., Mastrominas, M., & Yiannakouris, N. (2018). Adherence to the Mediterranean diet and IVF success rate among non-obese women attempting fertility. Human Reproduction, 33(3), 494-502.

21 Vujkovic M, de Vries JH, Lindemans J, Macklon NS, van der Spek PJ, Steegers EA, Steegers-Theunissen RP. The preconception Mediterranean dietary pattern in couples undergoing in vitro fertilization/ intracytoplasmic sperm injection treatment increases the chance of pregnancy.Fertil Steril. 2010 Nov;94(6):2096-101 ("Vujkovic 2010").

22 Ebisch IM, Peters WH, Thomas CM, Wetzels AM, Peer PG, Steegers-Theunissen RP. Homocysteine, glutathione and related thiols affect fertility parameters in the (sub)fertile couple.Hum Reprod. 2006 Jul;21(7):1725-33.

23 Chakrabarty P, Goswami SK, Rajani S, Sharma S, Kabir SN, Chakravarty B, Jana K. Recurrent pregnancy loss in polycystic ovary syndrome: role of hyperhomocysteinemia and insulin resistance. PLoS One. 2013 May 21;8(5):e64446; Wouters MG, Boers GH, Blom HJ, Trijbels FJ, Thomas CM, Borm GF, Steegers-Theunissen RP, Eskes TK. Hyperhomocysteinemia: a

risk factor in women with unexplained recurrent early pregnancy loss. Fertil Steril. 1993 Nov;60(5):820-5.

24 Koloverou, E., Panagiotakos, D. B., Pitsavos, C., Chrysohoou, C., Georgousopoulou, E. N., Grekas, A.,... & Stefanadis, C. (2016). Adherence to Mediterranean diet and 10-year incidence (2002–2012) of diabetes: correlations with inflammatory and oxidative stress biomarkers in the ATTICA cohort study. Diabetes/ metabolism research and reviews, 32(1), 73-81.
Arouca, A., Michels, N., Moreno, L. A., González-Gil, E. M., Marcos, A., Gómez, S.,... & Gottrand, F. (2018). Associations between a Mediterranean diet pattern and inflammatory biomarkers in European adolescents. European journal of nutrition, 57(5), 1747-1760.

25 Ronnenberg AG, Venners SA, Xu X, Chen C, Wang L, Guang W, Huang A, Wang X. Preconception B-vitamin and homocysteine status, conception, and early pregnancy loss.Am J Epidemiol. 2007 Aug 1;166(3):304-12.

26 Vujkovic 2010

27 Mirabi, P., Chaichi, M. J., Esmaeilzadeh, S., Jorsaraei, S. G. A., Bijani, A., Ehsani, M., & hashemi Karooee, S. F. (2017). The role of fatty acids on ICSI outcomes: a prospective cohort study. Lipids in health and disease, 16(1), 18
Moran, L. J., Tsagareli, V., Noakes, M., & Norman, R. (2016). Altered preconception fatty acid intake is associated with improved pregnancy rates in overweight and obese women undertaking in vitro fertilisation. Nutrients, 8(1), 10
Chiu, Y. H., Karmon, A. E., Gaskins, A. J., Arvizu, M., Williams, P. L., Souter, I.,... & EARTH Study Team. (2017). Serum omega-3 fatty acids and treatment outcomes among women undergoing assisted reproduction. Human Reproduction, 33(1), 156-165.)
Hammiche F, Vujkovic M, Wijburg W, de Vries JH, Macklon NS, Laven JS, Steegers-Theunissen RP. Increased preconception omega-3 polyunsaturated fatty acid intake improves embryo morphology. Fertil Steril. 2011 Apr;95(5):1820-3.

28 Hammiche F, Vujkovic M, Wijburg W, de Vries JH, Macklon NS, Laven JS, Steegers-Theunissen RP. Increased preconception omega-3 polyunsaturated fatty acid intake improves embryo morphology. Fertil Steril. 2011 Apr;95(5):1820-3.

29 Chiu, Y. H., Karmon, A. E., Gaskins, A. J., Arvizu, M., Williams, P. L., Souter, I.,... & EARTH Study Team. (2017). Serum omega-3 fatty acids and treatment outcomes among women undergoing assisted reproduction. Human Reproduction, 33(1), 156-165.)

30  Gaskins, A. J., Sundaram, R., Louis, B., Germaine, M., & Chavarro, J. E. (2018). Seafood Intake, Sexual Activity, and Time to Pregnancy. The Journal of Clinical Endocrinology & Metabolism.

31  Wise, L. A., Wesselink, A. K., Tucker, K. L., Saklani, S., Mikkelsen, E. M., Cueto, H.,...& Rothman, K. J. (2017). Dietary Fat Intake and Fecundability in 2 Preconception Cohort Studies. American journal of epidemiology, 187(1), 60-74.

32  Karayiannis, D., Kontogianni, M. D., Mendorou, C., Mastrominas, M., & Yiannakouris, N. (2018). Adherence to the Mediterranean diet and IVF success rate among non-obese women attempting fertility. Human Reproduction, 33(3), 494-502.

33  Matorras, R., Ruiz, J. I., Mendoza, R., Ruiz, N., Sanjurjo, P., & Rodriguez-Escudero, F. J. (1998). Fatty acid composition of fertilization-failed human oocytes. Human reproduction (Oxford, England), 13(8), 2227-2230.
    Aardema, H., Vos, P. L., Lolicato, F., Roelen, B. A., Knijn, H. M., Vaandrager, A. B.,...& Gadella, B. M. (2011). Oleic acid prevents detrimental effects of saturated fatty acids on bovine oocyte developmental competence. Biology of reproduction, 85(1), 62-69.

34  Mirabi, P., Chaichi, M. J., Esmaeilzadeh, S., Jorsaraei, S. G. A., Bijani, A., Ehsani, M., & hashemi Karooee, S. F. (2017). The role of fatty acids on ICSI outcomes: a prospective cohort study. Lipids in health and disease, 16(1), 18.

35  Moran, L. J., Tsagareli, V., Noakes, M., & Norman, R. (2016). Altered preconception fatty acid intake is associated with improved pregnancy rates in overweight and obese women undertaking in vitro fertilisation. Nutrients, 8(1), 10.

36  Mirabi, P., Chaichi, M. J., Esmaeilzadeh, S., Jorsaraei, S. G. A., Bijani, A., Ehsani, M., & hashemi Karooee, S. F. (2017). The role of fatty acids on ICSI outcomes: a prospective cohort study. Lipids in health and disease, 16(1), 18.

37  Braga, D. P. A. F., Halpern, G., Setti, A. S., Figueira, R. C. S., Iaconelli Jr, A., & Borges Jr, E. (2015). The impact of food intake and social habits on embryo quality and the likelihood of blastocyst formation. Reproductive biomedicine online, 31(1), 30-38.

38  Parisi, F., Rousian, M., Huijgen, N. A., Koning, A. H. J., Willemsen, S. P., de Vries, J. H. M.,...& Steegers–Theunissen, R. P. M. (2017). Periconceptional maternal 'high fish and olive oil, low meat' dietary pattern is associated with increased embryonic growth: The Rotterdam Periconceptional Cohort (Predict) Study. Ultrasound in Obstetrics & Gynecology, 50(6), 709-716.

39  Arouca, A., Michels, N., Moreno, L. A., González-Gil, E. M., Marcos, A., Gómez, S.,...& Gottrand, F. (2018). Associations between a Mediterranean diet pattern and inflammatory biomarkers in European adolescents. European journal of nutrition, 57(5), 1747-1760.

40  Wagner, M. M., Jukema, J. W., Hermes, W., le Cessie, S., de Groot, C. J., Bakker, J. A.,...& Bloemenkamp, K. W. (2018). Assessment of novel cardiovascular biomarkers in women with a history of recurrent miscarriage. Pregnancy hypertension, 11, 129-135. See also: Ahmed, S. K., Mahmood, N., Malalla, Z. H., Alsobyani, F. M., Al-Kiyumi, I. S., & Almawi, W. Y. (2015). C-reactive protein gene variants associated with recurrent pregnancy loss independent of CRP serum levels: a case-control study. Gene, 569(1), 136-140.

Kushnir, V. A., Solouki, S., Sarig–Meth, T., Vega, M. G., Albertini, D. F., Darmon, S. K.,...& Gleicher, N. (2016). Systemic inflammation and autoimmunity in women with chronic endometritis. American Journal of Reproductive Immunology, 75(6), 672-677.

41  Lahoz, C., Castillo, E., Mostaza, J. M., de Dios, O., Salinero-Fort, M. A., González-Alegre, T.,...& Sabín, C. (2018). Relationship of the adherence to a mediterranean diet and its main components with CRP levels in the Spanish population. Nutrients, 10(3), 379. Arouca, A., Michels, N, Moreno, L. A, González Gil, E. M., Marcos, A., Gómez, S.,...& Gottrand, F. (2018). Associations between a Mediterranean diet pattern and inflammatory biomarkers in European adolescents. European journal of nutrition, 57(5), 1747-1760.

42  Marziali, M., Venza, M., Lazzaro, S., Lazzaro, A., Micossi, C., & Stolfi, V. M. (2012). Gluten-free diet: a new strategy for management of painful endometriosis related symptoms? Minerva chirurgica, 67(6), 499-504. Marziali, M., & Capozzolo, T. (2015). Role of Gluten-Free Diet in the Management of Chronic Pelvic Pain of Deep Infiltranting Endometriosis. Journal of minimally invasive gynecology, 22(6), S51-S52.

43  Jensen TK, Hjollund NH, Henriksen TB, Scheike T, Kolstad H, Giwercman A, Ernst E, Bonde JP, Skakkebaek NE, Olsen J. Does moderate alcohol consumption affect fertility? Follow up study among couples planning first pregnancy. BMJ. 1998 Aug 22;317(7157):505-10 ("Jensen 1998a");

44 Juhl M, Nyboe Andersen AM, Grønbaek M, Olsen J. Moderate alcohol consumption and waiting time to pregnancy. Hum Reprod. 2001 Dec;16(12):2705-9;

45 Mikkelsen, E. M., Riis, A. H., Wise, L. A., Hatch, E. E., Rothman, K. J., Cueto, H. T., & Sørensen, H. T. (2016). Alcohol consumption and fecundability: prospective Danish cohort study. bmj, 354, i4262.

46 Rossi BV, Berry KF, Hornstein MD, Cramer DW, Ehrlich S, Missmer SA. Effect of alcohol consumption on in vitro fertilization. Obstet Gynecol. 2011 Jan;117(1):136-42.

47 Nicolau, P., Miralpeix, E., Sola, I., Carreras, R., & Checa, M. A. (2014). Alcohol consumption and in vitro fertilization: a review of the literature. Gynecological Endocrinology, 30(11), 759-763.

48 Vittrup, I., Petersen, G. L., Kamper-Jørgensen, M., Pinborg, A., & Schmidt, L. (2017). Male and female alcohol consumption and live birth after assisted reproductive technology treatment: A nationwide register-based cohort study. Reproductive biomedicine online, 35(2), 152-160.

49 Abadia, L., Chiu, Y. H., Williams, P. L., Toth, T. L., Souter, I., Hauser, R.,... & EARTH Study Team. (2017). The association between pre-treatment maternal alcohol and caffeine intake and outcomes of assisted reproduction in a prospectively followed cohort. Human Reproduction, 32(9), 1846-1854.

50 Avalos, L. A., Roberts, S. C., Kaskutas, L. A., Block, G., & Li, D. K. (2014). Volume and type of alcohol during early pregnancy and the risk of miscarriage. Substance use & misuse, 49(11), 1437-1445.

51 Gaskins, A. J., Rich-Edwards, J. W., Williams, P. L., Toth, T. L., Missmer, S. A., & Chavarro, J. E. (2015). Prepregnancy Low to Moderate Alcohol Intake Is Not Associated with Risk of Spontaneous Abortion or Stillbirth-3. The Journal of nutrition, 146(4), 799-805.

52 Ford, H. B., & Schust, D. J. (2009). Recurrent pregnancy loss: etiology, diagnosis, and therapy. Reviews in obstetrics and gynecology, 2(2), 76.

53 Gaskins, A. J., Rich-Edwards, J. W., Williams, P. L., Toth, T. L., Missmer, S. A., & Chavarro, J. E. (2018). Pre-pregnancy caffeine and caffeinated beverage intake and risk of spontaneous abortion. European journal of nutrition, 57(1), 107-117.

54 Chen, L. W., Wu, Y., Neelakantan, N., Chong, M. F. F., Pan, A., & van Dam, R. M. (2016). Maternal caffeine intake during pregnancy and risk of pregnancy loss: a categorical and dose–response meta-analysis of prospective studies. Public health nutrition, 19(7), 1233-1244.

55  Huang H, Hansen KR, Factor-Litvak P, Carson SA, Guzick DS, Santoro N, Diamond MP, Eisenberg E, Zhang H; National Institute of Child Health and Human Development Cooperative Reproductive Medicine Network. Predictors of pregnancy and live birth after insemination in couples with unexplained or male-factor infertility. Fertil Steril. 2012 Apr;97(4):959-67.

56  Al-Saleh I, El-Doush I, Grisellhi B, Coskun S. The effect of caffeine consumption on the success rate of pregnancy as well various performance parameters of in-vitro fertilization treatment. Med Sci Monit. 2010 Dec;16(12):CR598-605.

## Chapter 14: The Other Half of the Equation: Sperm Quality

1  Esteves SC, Agarwal A. Novel concepts in male infertility. Int Braz J Urol. 2011 Jan-Feb;37(1):5-15.

2  Kumar K, Deka D, Singh A, Mitra DK, Vanitha BR, Dada R. Predictive value of DNA integrity analysis in idiopathic recurrent pregnancy loss following spontaneous conception. J Assist Reprod Genet. 2012 Sep;29(9):861-7.

3  Jayasena, C. N., Radia, U. K., Figueiredo, M., Revill, L. F., Dimakopoulou, A., Osagie, M.,...& Dhillo, W. S. (2019). Reduced Testicular Steroidogenesis and Increased Semen Oxidative Stress in Male Partners as Novel Markers of Recurrent Miscarriage. Clinical Chemistry, 65(1), 161-169.

4  Simon, L., Zini, A., Dyachenko, A., Ciampi, A., & Carrell, D. T. (2017). A systematic review and meta-analysis to determine the effect of sperm DNA damage on in vitro fertilization and intracytoplasmic sperm injection outcome. Asian journal of andrology, 19(1), 80.

5  Siddighi S, Chan CA, Patton WC, Jacobson JD, Chan PJ: Male age and sperm necrosis in assisted reproductive technologies. Urol Int. 2007; 9: 231-4 ("Siddighi 2007").

6  Singh NP, Muller CH, Berger RE. Effects of age on DNA double-strand breaks and apoptosis in human sperm. Fertil Steril. 2003 Dec;80(6):1420-30;
Wyrobek AJ, Eskenazi B, Young S, Arnheim N, Tiemann-Boege I, Jabs EW, Glaser RL, Pearson FS, Evenson D. Advancing age has differential effects on DNA damage, chromatin integrity, gene mutations, and aneuploidies in sperm. Proc Natl Acad Sci U S A. 2006 Jun 20;103(25):9601-6;
Schmid TE, Eskenazi B, Baumgartner A, Marchetti F, Young S, Weldon R, Anderson D, Wyrobek AJ. The effects of male age on

sperm DNA damage in healthy non-smokers. Hum Reprod. 2007 Jan;22(1):180-7.

7   Moskovtsev SI, Willis J, Mullen JB: Age-related decline in sperm deoxyribonucleic acid integrity in patients evaluated for male infertility. Fertil Steril. 2006; 85: 496-9.

8   Wyrobek AJ, Aardema M, Eichenlaub-Ritter U, Ferguson L, Marchetti F: Mechanisms and targets involved in maternal and paternal age effects on numerical aneuploidy. Environ Mol Mutagen. 1996; 28: 254-64.

9   Robinson L, Gallos ID, Conner SJ, Rajkhowa M, Miller D, Lewis S, Kirkman-Brown J, Coomarasamy A. The effect of sperm DNA fragmentation on miscarriage rates: a systematic review and meta-analysis. Hum Reprod. 2012 Oct;27(10):2908-17 ("Robinson 2012").

10  Johnson L, Petty CS, Porter JC, Neaves WB: Germ cell degeneration during postprophase of meiosis and serum concentrations of gonadotropins in young adult and older adult men. Biol Reprod. 1984; 31: 779-84.18;
Plastira K, Msaouel P, Angelopoulou R, Zanioti K, Plastiras A, Pothos A, Bolaris S, Paparisteidis N, Mantas D: The effects of age on DNA fragmentation, chromatin packaging and conventional semen parameters in spermatozoa of oligoasthenoteratozoospermic patients. J Assist Reprod Genet. 2007; 24: 437-43.
Siddighi 2007

11  Misell LM, Holochwost D, Boban D, Santi N, Shefi N, Hellerstein MK, Turek PJ: A stable isotope-mass spectrometric method for measuring human spermatogenesis kinetics in vivo. J Urol. 2006; 175: 242-6

12  Auger J, Eustache F, Andersen AG, Irvine DS, Jørgensen N, Skakkebaek NE, Suominen J, Toppari J, Vierula M, Jouannet P: Sperm morphological defects related to environment, lifestyle and medical history of 1001 male partners of pregnant women from four European cities. Hum Reprod. 2001; 16: 2710-7.

13  Armstrong JS, Rajasekaran M, Chamulitrat W, Gatti P, Hellstrom WJ, Sikka SC. Characterization of reactive oxygen species induced effects on human spermatozoa movement and energy metabolism. Free Radic. Biol. Med. 1999; 26: 869–80. 12
Kodama H, Yamaguchi R, Fukuda J, Kasai H, Tanaka T. Increased oxidative deoxyribonucleic acid damage in the spermatozoa of infertile male patients. Fertil. Steril. 1997; 68: 519–24. 13
Barroso G, Morshedi M, Oehninger S. Analysis of DNA fragmentation, plasma membrane translocation of

phosphatidylserine and oxidative stress in human spermatozoa. Hum. Reprod. 2000; 15: 1338–44.

14  Mahfouz R, Sharma R, Thiyagarajan A, Kale V, Gupta S, Sabanegh E, Agarwal A. Semen characteristics and sperm DNA fragmentation in infertile men with low and high levels of seminal reactive oxygen species. Fertil Steril. 2010 Nov;94(6):2141-6.

15  Wong EW, Cheng CY. Impacts of environmental toxicants on male reproductive dysfunction. Trends Pharmacol Sci. 2011 May;32(5):290-9.

16  Esteves 2012.

17  Meseguer M, Martínez-Conejero JA, O'Connor JE, Pellicer A, Remohí J, Garrido N. The significance of sperm DNA oxidation in embryo development and reproductive outcome in an oocyte donation program: a new model to study a male infertility prognostic factor. Fertil Steril. 2008 May;89(5):1191-9.

18  Ross C, Morriss A, Khairy M, Khalaf Y, Braude P, Coomarasamy A, El-Toukhy T. A systematic review of the effect of oral antioxidants on male infertility. Reprod Biomed Online. 2010 Jun;20(6):711-23 ("Ross 2010").
    Showell MG, Brown J, Yazdani A, Stankiewicz MT, Hart RJ. Antioxidants for male subfertility. Cochrane Database of Systematic Reviews (Online) 2011;11:CD007411 ("Showell 2011"); Robinson 2012.

19  Showell 2011

20  Showell 2011.

21  Greco E, Romano S, Iacobelli M, Ferrero S, Baroni E, Minasi MG, Ubaldi F, Rienzi L, Tesarik J. ICSI in cases of sperm DNA damage: beneficial effect of oral antioxidant treatment. Hum Reprod. 2005 Sep;20(9):2590-4 ("Greco 2005b").

22  Ross C, Morriss A, Khairy M, Khalaf Y, Braude P, Coomarasamy A, El-Toukhy T. A systematic review of the effect of oral antioxidants on male infertility. Reprod Biomed Online. 2010 Jun;20(6):711-23.

23  Schmid TE, Eskenazi B, Marchetti F, Young S, Weldon RH, Baumgartner A, Anderson D, Wyrobek AJ. Micronutrients intake is associated with improved sperm DNA quality in older men. Fertil Steril. 2012 Nov;98(5):1130-7.e1

24  Kos, B. J., Leemaqz, S. Y., McCormack, C. D., Andraweera, P. H., Furness, D. L., Roberts, C. T., & Dekker, G. A. (2018). The association of parental methylenetetrahydrofolate reductase polymorphisms (MTHFR 677C> T and 1298A> C) and fetal loss:

a case–control study in South Australia. The Journal of Maternal-Fetal & Neonatal Medicine, 1-6

Vanilla, S., Dayanand, C. D., Kotur, P. F., Kutty, M. A., & Vegi, P. K. (2015). Evidence of paternal N5, N10-methylenetetrahydrofolate reductase (MTHFR) C677T gene polymorphism in couples with recurrent spontaneous abortions (RSAs) in Kolar District-A South West of India. Journal of clinical and diagnostic research: JCDR, 9(2), BC15.

Govindaiah, V., Naushad, S. M., Prabhakara, K., Krishna, P. C., & Devi, A. R. R. (2009). Association of parental hyperhomocysteinemia and C677T Methylene tetrahydrofolate reductase (MTHFR) polymorphism with recurrent pregnancy loss. Clinical biochemistry, 42(4-5), 380-386.

25  Govindaiah, V., Naushad, S. M., Prabhakara, K., Krishna, P. C., & Devi, A. R. R. (2009). Association of parental hyperhomocysteinemia and C677T Methylene tetrahydrofolate reductase (MTHFR) polymorphism with recurrent pregnancy loss. Clinical biochemistry, 42(4-5), 380-386.

26  Mancini A, De Marinis L, Oradei A, Hallgass ME, Conte G, Pozza D, Littarru GP. Coenzyme Q10 concentrations in normal and pathological human seminal fluid. J Androl. 1994 Nov-Dec;15(6):591-4.

27  Lafuente R, González-Comadrán M, Solà I, López G, Brassesco M, Carreras R, Checa MA. Coenzyme Q10 and male infertility: a meta-analysis. J Assist Reprod Genet. 2013 Sep;30(9):1147-56; Nadjarzadeh A, Shidfar F, Amirjannati N, Vafa MR, Motevalian SA, Gohari MR, Nazeri Kakhki SA, Akhondi MM, Sadeghi MR. Effect of Coenzyme Q10 supplementation on antioxidant enzymes activity and oxidative stress of seminal plasma: a double-blind randomised clinical trial. Andrologia. 2013 Jan 7 ("Nadjarzadeh 2013"). Balercia 2009, Safarinejad 12.

28  Abad C, Amengual MJ, Gosálvez J, Coward K, Hannaoui N, Benet J, García-Peiró A, Prats J. Effects of oral antioxidant treatment upon the dynamics of human sperm DNA fragmentation and subpopulations of sperm with highly degraded DNA. Andrologia. 2013 Jun;45(3):211-6.

29  Nadjarzadeh 2013.

30  Tirabassi, G., Vignini, A., Tiano, L., Buldreghini, E., Brugè, F., Silvestri, S.,...& Balercia, G. (2015). Protective effects of coenzyme Q 10 and aspartic acid on oxidative stress and DNA damage in subjects affected by idiopathic asthenozoospermia. Endocrine, 49(2), 549-552.

31  Safarinejad MR, Safarinejad S, Shafiei N, Safarinejad S. Effects of the reduced form of coenzyme Q10 (ubiquinol) on semen parameters in men with idiopathic infertility: a double-blind, placebo controlled, randomized study. J Urol. 2012 Aug;188(2):526-31.
32  Haghighian, H. K., Haidari, F., Mohammadi-asl, J., & Dadfar, M. (2015). Randomized, triple-blind, placebo-controlled clinical trial examining the effects of alpha-lipoic acid supplement on the spermatogram and seminal oxidative stress in infertile men. Fertility and sterility, 104(2), 318-324.
33  Salas-Huetos, A., Rosique-Esteban, N., Becerra-Tomás, N., Vizmanos, B., Bulló, M., & Salas-Salvadó, J. (2018). The Effect of Nutrients and Dietary Supplements on Sperm Quality Parameters: A Systematic Review and Meta-Analysis of Randomized Clinical Trials. Advances in Nutrition, 9(6), 833-848.
    Martínez-Soto, J. C., Domingo, J. C., Cordobilla, B., Nicolás, M., Fernández, L., Albero, P.,...& Landeras, J. (2016). Dietary supplementation with docosahexaenoic acid (DHA) improves seminal antioxidant status and decreases sperm DNA fragmentation. Systems biology in reproductive medicine, 62(6), 387-395.
34  Martínez-Soto, J. C., Domingo, J. C., Cordobilla, B., Nicolás, M., Fernández, L., Albero, P.,...& Landeras, J. (2016). Dietary supplementation with docosahexaenoic acid (DHA) improves seminal antioxidant status and decreases sperm DNA fragmentation. Systems biology in reproductive medicine, 62(6), 387-395.
35  Salas-Huetos, A., Rosique-Esteban, N., Becerra-Tomás, N., Vizmanos, B., Bulló, M., & Salas-Salvadó, J. (2018). The Effect of Nutrients and Dietary Supplements on Sperm Quality Parameters: A Systematic Review and Meta-Analysis of Randomized Clinical Trials. Advances in Nutrition, 9(6), 833-848.
36  Vessey, W., McDonald, C., Virmani, A., Almeida, P., Jayasena, C., & Ramsay, J. (2016, October). Levels of reactive oxygen species (ROS) in the seminal plasma predicts the effectiveness of L-carnitine to improve sperm function in men with infertility. In Society for Endocrinology BES 2016 (Vol. 44). BioScientifica.
37  Sofimajidpour, H., Ghaderi, E., & Ganji, O. (2016). Comparison of the effects of varicocelectomy and oral L-carnitine on sperm parameters in infertile men with varicocele. Journal of clinical and diagnostic research: JCDR, 10(4), PC07.
38  Balercia, G., Regoli, F., Armeni, T., Koverech, A., Mantero, F., & Boscaro, M. (2005). Placebo-controlled double-blind randomized trial on the use of L-carnitine, L-acetylcarnitine, or combined

L-carnitine and L-acetylcarnitine in men with idiopathic asthenozoospermia. Fertility and sterility, 84(3), 662-671. Zhou, X., Liu, F., & Zhai, S. D. (2007). Effect of L-carnitine and/or L-acetyl-carnitine in nutrition treatment for male infertility: a systematic review. Asia Pacific journal of clinical nutrition, 16(S1), 383-390.

39  Young SS, Eskenazi B, Marchetti FM, Block G, Wyrobek AJ. The association of folate, zinc and antioxidant intake with sperm aneuploidy in healthy non-smoking men. Hum Reprod. 2008 May;23(5):1014-22 ("Young 2008");
Mendiola J, Torres-Cantero AM, Vioque J, Moreno-Grau JM, Ten J, Roca M, Moreno-Grau S, Bernabeu R. A low intake of antioxidant nutrients is associated with poor semen quality in patients attending fertility clinics. Fertil Steril. 2010;11:1128–1133.
Silver EW, Eskenazi B, Evenson DP, Block G, Young S, Wyrobek AJ. Effect of antioxidant intake on sperm chromatin stability in healthy nonsmoking men. J Androl. 2005 Jul-Aug;26(4):550-6.

40  Braga DP, Halpern G, Figueira Rde C, Setti AS, Iaconelli A Jr, Borges E Jr. Food intake and social habits in male patients and its relationship to intracytoplasmic sperm injection outcomes. Fertil Steril. 2012 Jan;97(1):53-9.

41  Young 2008.

42  Schmid TE, Eskenazi B, Marchetti F, Young S, Weldon RH, Baumgartner A, Anderson D, Wyrobek AJ. Micronutrients intake is associated with improved sperm DNA quality in older men. Fertil Steril. 2012 Nov;98(5):1130-7.e1.

43  Gupta NP, Kumar R (2002) Lycopene therapy in idiopathic male infertility—a preliminary report. Int Urol Nephrol 34(3):369– 372.

44  Chiu, Y. H., Gaskins, A. J., Williams, P. L., Mendiola, J., Jørgensen, N., Levine, H.,... & Chavarro, J. E. (2016). Intake of Fruits and Vegetables with Low-to-Moderate Pesticide Residues Is Positively Associated with Semen-Quality Parameters among Young Healthy Men–3. The Journal of nutrition, 146(5), 1084-1092.

45  Salas-Huetos, A., Bulló, M., & Salas-Salvadó, J. (2017). Dietary patterns, foods and nutrients in male fertility parameters and fecundability: a systematic review of observational studies. Human reproduction update, 23(4), 371-389.

46  Gaur DS, Talekar MS, Pathak VP. Alcohol intake and cigarette smoking: Impact of two major lifestyle factors on male fertility. Indian J Pathol Microbiol. 2010;11:35–40.
Muthusami KR, Chinnaswamy P. Effect of chronic alcoholism on male fertility hormones and semen quality. Fertil Steril. 2005;11:919–924

47 Klonoff-Cohen H, Lam-Kruglick P, Gonzalez C. Effects of maternal and paternal alcohol consumption on the success rates of in vitro fertilization and gamete intrafallopian transfer. Fertil Steril. 2003;79:330–9.

48 Braga DP, Halpern G, Figueira Rde C, Setti AS, Iaconelli A Jr, Borges E Jr. Food intake and social habits in male patients and its relationship to intracytoplasmic sperm injection outcomes. Fertil Steril. 2012 Jan;97(1):53-9.

49 Koch OR, Pani G, Borrello S et al. Oxidative stress and antioxidant defenses in ethanol-induced cell injury. Mol Aspects Med. 2004; 25: 191–8.

50 Huang XF, Li Y, Gu YH, Liu M, Xu Y, Yuan Y, Sun F, Zhang HQ, Shi HJ. The effects of Di-(2-ethylhexyl)-phthalate exposure on fertilization and embryonic development in vitro and testicular genomic mutation in vivo. PLoS One. 2012;7(11):e50465; Pant N, Pant A, Shukla M, Mathur N, Gupta Y, Saxena D. Environmental and experimental exposure of phthalate esters: the toxicological consequence on human sperm. Hum Exp Toxicol. 2011 Jun;30(6):507-14; Duty S. M., Singh N. P., Silva M. J., Barr D. B., Brock J. W., Ryan L., Herrick R. F., Christiani D. C., Hauser R. 2003b. The relationship between environmental exposures to phthalates and DNA damage in human sperm using the neutral comet assay. Environ. Health Perspect. 111, 1164–1169. ("In conclusion, this study represents the first human data to demonstrate that urinary MEP, at environmental levels, is associated with increased DNA damage in sperm.")

51 Mendiola J, Meeker JD, Jørgensen N, Andersson AM, Liu F, Calafat AM, Redmon JB, Drobnis EZ, Sparks AE, Wang C, Hauser R, Swan SH. Urinary concentrations of di(2-ethylhexyl) phthalate metabolites and serum reproductive hormones: pooled analysis of fertile and infertile men. J Androl. 2012 May-Jun;33(3):488-98. Meeker J. D., Calafat A.M., Hauser R. Urinary metabolites of di(2-ethylhexyl) phthalate are associated with decreased steroid hormone levels in adult men.. J Androl. 2009 May–Jun; 30(3): 287–297.

52 Ferguson KK, Loch-Caruso R, Meeker JD. Urinary phthalate metabolites in relation to biomarkers of inflammation and oxidative stress: NHANES 1999-2006. Environ Res. 2011 Jul;111(5):718-26.

53 Buck Louis G.M., Sundaram R., Sweeney A., Schisterman E.F., Kannan K. Bisphenol A, phthalates and couple fecundity, the life study. Fertil. Steril. 2013 Sep; 100(3): S1.

54 Meeker JD, Ehrlich S, Toth TL, Wright DL, Calafat AM, Trisini AT, Ye X, Hauser R. Semen quality and sperm DNA damage in

relation to urinary bisphenol A among men from an infertility clinic. Reprod Toxicol. 2010 Dec;30(4):532-9.

55  Knez J, Kranvogl R, Breznik BP, Vončina E, Vlaisavljević V. Are urinary bisphenol A levels in men related to semen quality and embryo development after medically assisted reproduction? Fertil Steril. 2014 Jan;101(1):215-221.e5Li DK, Zhou Z, Miao M, He Y, Wang J, Ferber J, Herrinton LJ, Gao E, Yuan W. Urine bisphenol-A (BPA) level in relation to semen quality. Fertil Steril. 2011 Feb;95(2):625-30.e1-4.

56  Liu C, Duan W, Zhang L, Xu S, Li R, Chen C, He M, Lu Y, Wu H, Yu Z, Zhou Z. Bisphenol A exposure at an environmentally relevant dose induces meiotic abnormalities in adult male rats. Cell Tissue Res. 2014 Jan;355(1):223-32.

57  Wu HM, Lin-Tan DT, Wang ML, Huang HY, Lee CL, Wang HS, Soong YK, Lin JL. Lead level in seminal plasma may affect semen quality for men without occupational exposure to lead. Reprod Biol Endocrinol. 2012 Nov 8;10:91. Telisman S, Colak B, Pizent A, Jurasović J, Cvitković P. Reproductive toxicity of low-level lead exposure in men. Environ Res. 2007 Oct;105(2):256-66. Hernández-Ochoa I, García-Vargas G, López-Carrillo L, Rubio-Andrade M, Morán-Martínez J, Cebrián ME, Quintanilla-Vega B. Low lead environmental exposure alters semen quality and sperm chromatin condensation in northern Mexico. Reprod Toxicol. 2005 Jul-Aug; 20(2):221-8.

58  http://www.ewg.org/report/ewgs-water-filter-buying-guide

59  http://www.ewg.org/research/dirty-dozen-list-endocrine-disruptors

60  Sandhu RS, Wong TH, Kling CA, Chohan KR. In vitro effects of coital lubricants and synthetic and natural oils on sperm motility. Fertil Steril. 2014 Jan 23 [Epub ahead of print] ("Sandhu 2014"); Agarwal A, Deepinder F, Cocuzza M, Short RA, Evenson DP. Effect of vaginal lubricants on sperm motility and chromatin integrity: a prospective comparative study. Fertil Steril. 2008 Feb;89(2):375-9.

61  Mowat, A., Newton, C., Boothroyd, C., Demmers, K., & Fleming, S. (2014). The effects of vaginal lubricants on sperm function: an in vitro analysis. Journal of assisted reproduction and genetics, 31(3), 333-339.

62  Agarwal A, Deepinder F, Sharma RK, Ranga G, Li J. Effect of cell phone usage on semen analysis in men attending infertility clinic: An observational study. Fertil Steril. 2008;11:124–128

63  Agarwal A, Desai NR, Makker K, Varghese A, Mouradi R, Sabanegh E, Sharma R. Effects of radiofrequency electromagnetic

waves (RF-EMW) from cellular phones on human ejaculated semen: An in vitro pilot study. Fertil Steril. 2009;11:1318–1325.

64 Agarwal A, Singh A, Hamada A, Kesari K. Cell phones and male infertility: A review of recent innovations in technology and consequences. Int Braz J Urol. 2011;11:432–454.

65 Carlsen E, Andersson AM, Petersen JH, Skakkebaek NE. History of febrile illness and variation in semen quality. Hum. Reprod. 2003; 18: 2089–92.

66 Jung A, Leonhardt F, Schill W, Schuppe H. Influence of the type of undertrousers and physical activity on scrotal temperature. Hum Reprod. 2005;11:1022–1027

67 Tiemessen CH, Evers JL, Bots RS. Tight-fitting underwear and sperm quality. Lancet. 1996;11:1844–1845.

24953581R00194

Printed in Great Britain
by Amazon